SENSUAL MASSAGE

A Lover's Guide

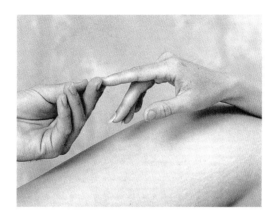

Susan Mumford

SENSUAL MASSAGE

A Lover's Guide

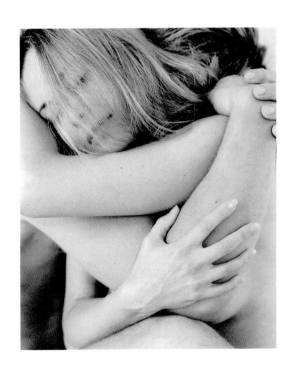

Susan Mumford

hamlyn

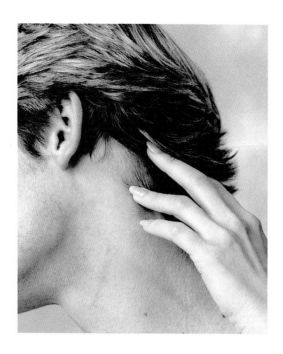

Photography by **Richard Truscott**

Art Editor **Trinity Fry**
Commissioning Editor **Sian Facer**
Art Director **Jacqui Small**
Editor **Susie Behar**
Production Controller **Sarah Rees**

First published in Great Britan in 1994 in hardback titled
The Sensual Touch: A Lover's Guide to Massage by Mitchell Beazley, an
imprint of Octopus Publishing Group Ltd

This paperback edition published by Hamlyn, an imprint of
Octopus Publishing Group Ltd
2-4 Heron Quays
London, E14 4JP

ISBN 0 600 60012 2

A CIP catalogue record for this book is available at the British Library

Printed and bound in Hong Kong by
Toppan Printing Co., (H.K.) Ltd.

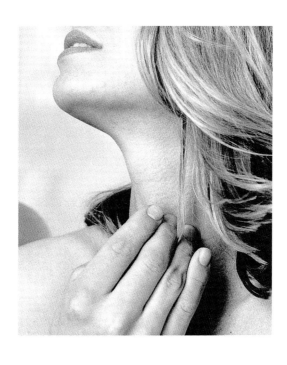

INTRODUCTION

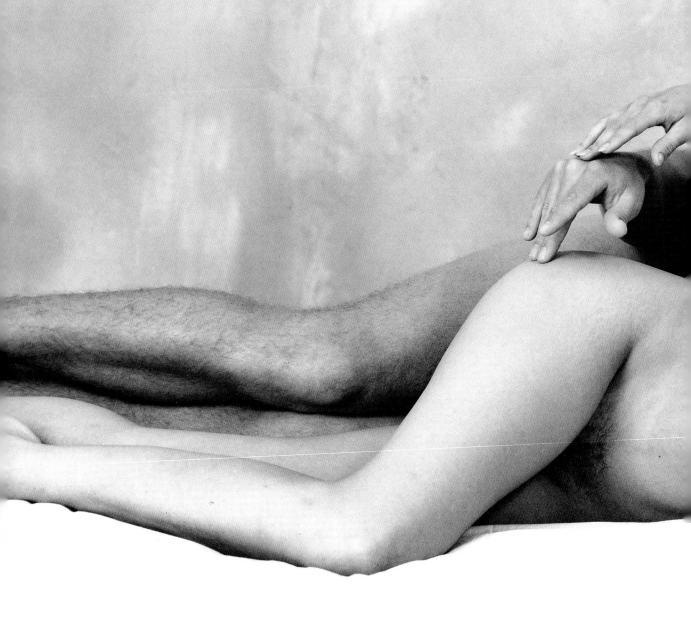

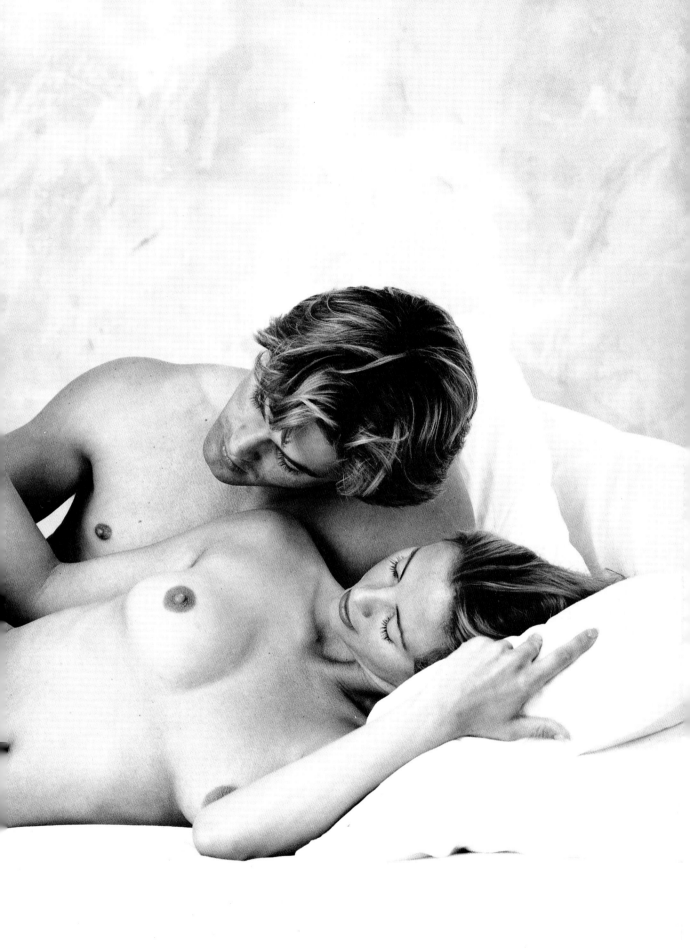

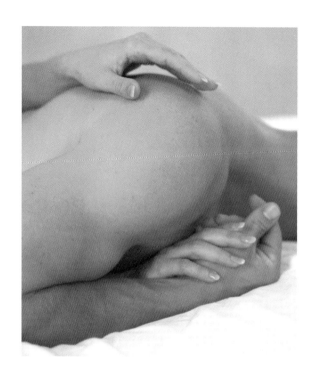

INTRODUCTION

*T*ouch. We love to touch. We are indeed tactile, sensual
beings. We perceive the world through our senses, and are
affected by what we receive. Sight, sound, taste, touch, smell – of
all the senses, touching perhaps affects us the most deeply.

Touch communicates, brings closeness, restores and arouses.
From infancy, we use touch to find out about the world, to
explore, reach out and confirm. Through touch we are able to
affirm or transform our relationships, find out information and
reveal or hide ourselves. Touch tells us who we are, it gives us a
sense of ourselves, allows us to make contact and feel we are not
alone. We use touch for pleasure, to bring relationships closer, to
comfort and accept. Instinctively we feel people as they walk into
a room – touch brings that contact closer, makes it real.

Our senses and feelings can give us balance and satisfaction.
They are an antidote to a thinking, technical world. In order to

find such a balance, we need to turn our focus to our senses, re-examine our surroundings, and see how they make us feel. We need to have an environment where we can feel, let go freely, where we can open up emotionally, receive pleasure and relax. Taking care to have around us objects that we like, inspiring shapes, softness, and curves. Paying attention to color, materials, scents and sounds, for each sensation conveys something to us.

In exploring the sensual world and our responses to it, we naturally increase our use of touch. Touching our surroundings, the people we encounter, those we are close to, and those we love. As lovers we are particularly vulnerable and open to each other – touch can give immense pleasure or cause physical pain.

The way that we, as lovers, touch defines the bond between us. Through sensuality we explore and find delight in each other, heightening both arousal and awareness. Pleasing each other, we bring the other closer, increasing our sense of loving and being loved.

Massage celebrates sensuality. It is an experience of giving and receiving, of exploring and opening to each other. It is a way of pleasing and relaxing, releasing stress and tension and creates a profound feeling of well-being. By giving massage we are caring for each other in a very real and loving way. In getting to know each other better, we increase the trust and sharing vital for

a loving relationship to thrive. The wonderful thing about massage is that it feels as good to give as to receive.

Massage can be used for simple relaxation – as a way of easing tired muscles, calming the mind, uplifting the spirit and restoring our natural energy. Having the ability to do this for our partner gives a special satisfaction, a feeling of confidence and warmth. For our partner, allowing a caring touch to discover and ease away stress and tensions is a statement of openness and their trust in us.

Intimate massage combines basic massage techniques, designed to relax and keep muscles healthy, with added sensual arousal and the spontaneity of loving touch. With sensual massage, each one pleasures and satisfies the other, creating an intimate, loving, two-way flow. There is no right way to do it, it depends on a shared experience. If our attention is on our partner, we will be concerned only with their happiness, and a tender sensitivity will develop. The beauty of a sensual, intimate massage is that it enhances our relationship, by increasing knowledge, vitality and joy.

The sensual massage in this book will take you about an hour to give. The relaxation massage takes about twenty minutes. If you don't have a full hour to spare, you can concentrate on one particular area of your partner's body, giving that area your full loving attention.

Preparing for MASSAGE

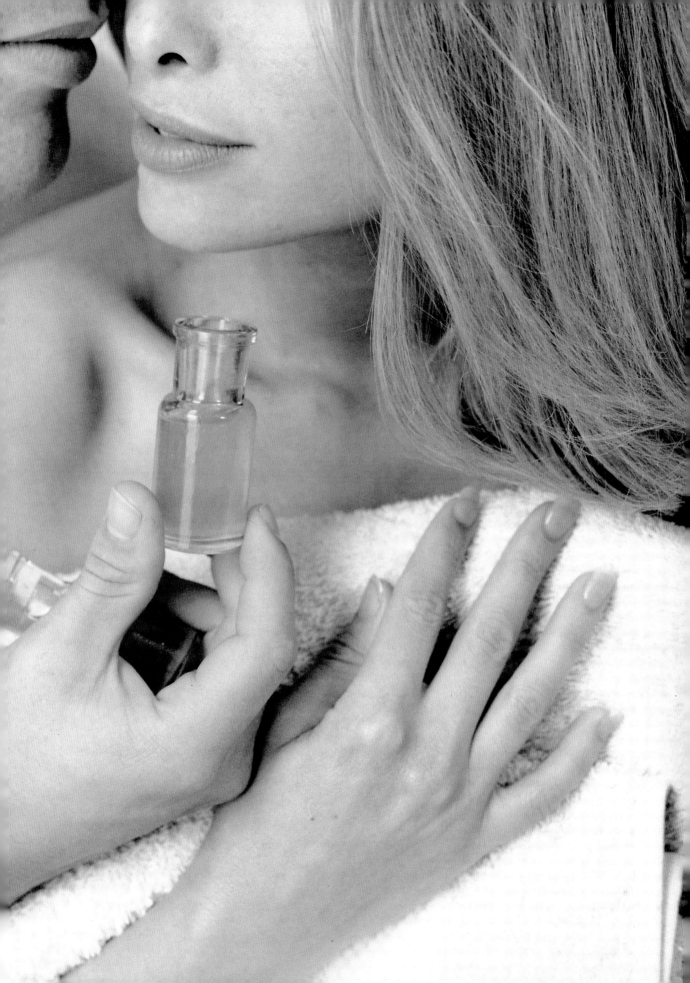

CREATING THE ENVIRONMENT

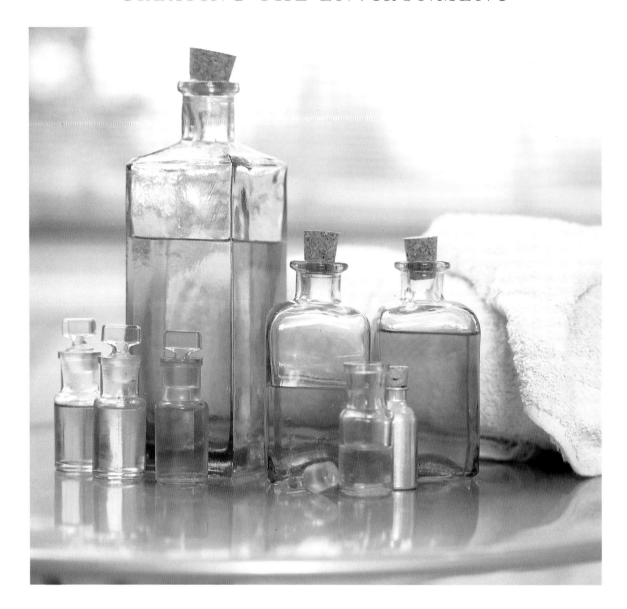

Preparing for a sensual massage can be a sensual experience in itself. It sets the mood, and the care and thought put into it will increase your enjoyment of the massage. Mixing and using oils can be extremely satisfying. There are various oils that you can use, and finding a combination that suits you is often just a matter of experimentation. The 'carrier' or 'base' oil is the basic oil used to allow the hands to glide freely over the skin. Grapeseed, a light vegetable oil without a heavy smell, is a very good carrier oil. Almond oil, a slightly sweeter, thicker oil, feels more luxurious on the skin. Oils of avocado and apricot are rich, nourishing oils, which may be added to make a mixture fuller. Oil of jojoba is a beautiful, more expensive oil, which is particularly good for massaging the face.

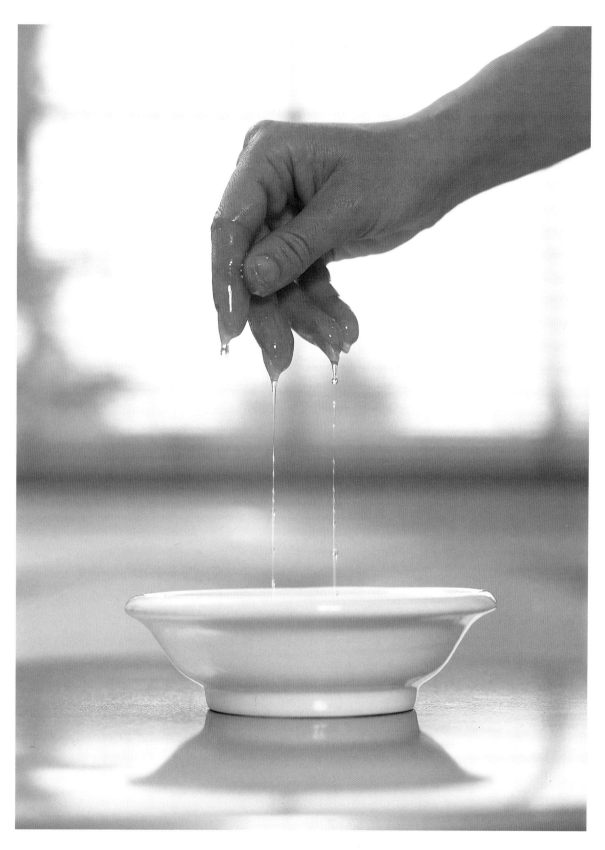

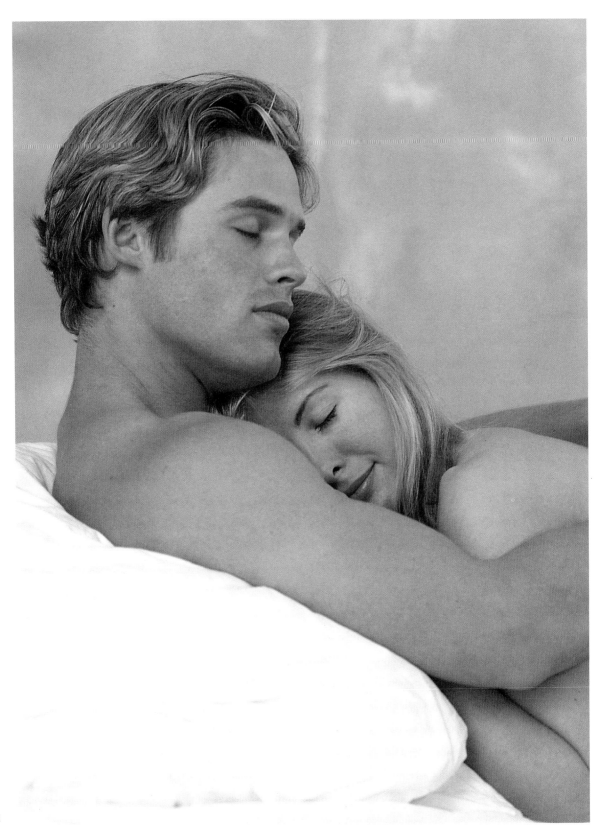

Another group of oils, essential oils, are added to the carrier oil to enhance the effect of massage. Containing the essential nature of a plant, they are extremely potent, and you need only use a few drops. Traditionally essential oils are used for the treatment of various conditions and they should not be used directly on the skin. For example, for relaxation, use lavender, a particularly useful, fresh, healing oil, or chamomile, which has a calming, sedative effect. In order to get to know them, try them separately at first, mixing a couple of drops into some oil. For heightening sensual arousal, try oils known as aphrodisiacs – sandalwood, a woody, sedating, eastern scent; patchouli, a more stimulating, sweet, dark odor; or ylang ylang, which has an euphoric, sweet, floral smell. Experiment with these oils and see which ones attract you. Perhaps the most beautiful of oils, and also the most expensive, are delicate neroli (orange blossom), which sedates; exotic jasmine, which uplifts; and luxurious, soothing oil of rose. Also

reputed to have aphrodisiacal properties, these are evocative, irresistibly heady scents. On pages 122-123 you will find a list of oils and their properties and some recipes for you to try out. Although mixing can be extremely satisfying, you can if you prefer, buy ready mixed oils.

There are various oils that you can use, and finding a combination that suits you is often just a matter of experimentation. You can make up as much as you like. If you start with 1floz (28ml) of base oil you will make enough oil for about four massages. The ratio you should remember is use up to, but not more than, 12 drops of essential oil per 1floz (28ml) of base oil. For the massage you can use a shallow dish in which to put some oil, or use a small bottle with a stopper. If you are planning to massage frequently, you could prepare a mixture by filling 1 or 2floz (28 or 54ml) glass bottles. If you add an optional teaspoon of wheat germ oil the mixture is preserved for a longer period.

relaxation

Before starting a massage it is important to tune into how you and your partner feel. Take all the time you need to relax together. When you are ready, try some gentle breathing to relax your mind and body. Lying on your back, knees bent, place your hands on your abdomen (top right). Simply allow your body to breathe naturally, feeling the rise and fall of your hands. After five or ten minutes, move and let each part of your body relax in turn. Then drawing your knees up to your chest, spread your arms, and slowly lower your left leg, and then your right leg, to the floor (bottom right). Next do this in reverse. This gives a wonderful stretch but does not strain.

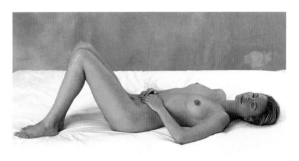

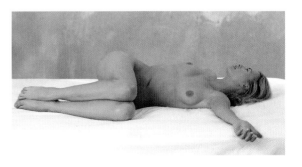

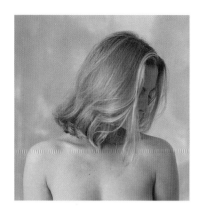 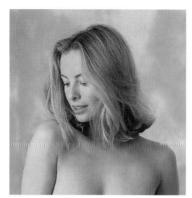

head and shoulders

Standing or sitting with your spine straight, drop your head forwards onto your chest. Now, very slowly, start circling your head round to the left. Let your head roll smoothly, making the circle generous, without any strain. Continue round to the right, then roll the other way, completing the circle at your chest. Raise your head slowly. Then, roll each shoulder in turn, slowly and evenly, focusing only on that movement.

After mixing up the oils it is important to make sure you have everything you need before beginning massage, so that you can give your full attention to your partner. The surface on which you massage should be comfortable but firm, giving your partner's body full support. You may need towels for warmth, and pillows to raise your partner's body. Have a supply of tissues, some water, and containers for the oil. Check to make sure the containers are well-balanced as it is extremely easy to knock them over as you move.

Before giving a massage, it is important also to prepare yourself. Never give a massage if you are tired. The contact between you and your partner becomes so close that almost your very thoughts can be sensed. Take time with your partner to gently relax your body. Allow your mind to clear, let go of any preoccupations, focusing your thoughts on your partner and yourself. Gentle breathing and body sensing, followed by muscle relaxation, help increase your inner balance. In order to relax the spine and release any neck or shoulder tension, follow the simple but effective movements shown here. Use the floor to give you support, and keep each action precise, focusing your mind entirely on the sensation, feeling your joints and muscles flow. You and your partner can do these exercises together or you can ask your partner to watch you, giving you help through feedback or touch. After the exercises, ask your partner to gently massage your neck and shoulders before you start, so you will have received before you give.

Finally, be creative with your room. Turn it into a sensual retreat, filling it with things you enjoy. Make sure it is warm, the lighting is soft, and that you will not be disturbed.

spine

To relax the spine, sit on your heels, your forehead on the floor. Now slowly start uncurling your spine, one vertebra at a time, until you reach a sitting position. Your lower back works first, and your head comes last, rolling up evenly through the spine.

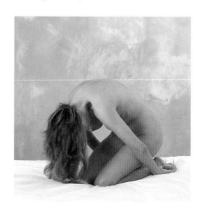

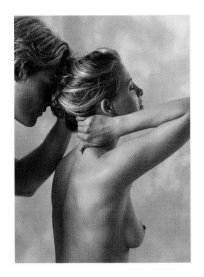

self-massage

To relax the neck muscles, you can use some simple self-massage. Hold your hand over the back of your neck, arching in the middle to avoid the spine, with the heel of your hand on one side and your fingertips on the other. Now by raising the arch of your hand, bring your fingertips and heel toward each other, gently working and squeezing the muscles on either side of your spine. With a rhythmic motion, work up your neck muscles to the base of your skull, where a lot of tension collects. Spend some time here and then work back down again. Use a pressure that feels comfortable. Drop your head slightly to open your neck muscles, slowly straightening as you reach the base of your skull.

shoulder massage

To ease your neck and shoulders, ask your partner to massage them for you. Your partner's fingers should be placed over your shoulders, without squeezing, so the thumbs are free to gently knead and press. The thumbs can circle, press and squeeze the muscles, starting about an inch out from the spine on either side. From here the movement continues, squeezing and lifting, out along the top of the shoulders. Returning to the spine, your partner should continue the movement downwards, keeping the same position of the hands. As your partner feels knots and tension, he should pay them special attention. It feels particularly good to be massaged between the shoulder blades.

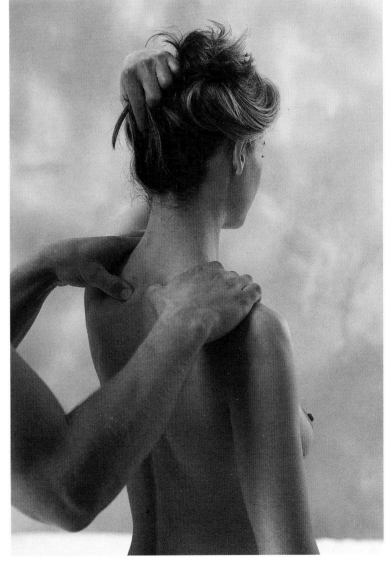

17

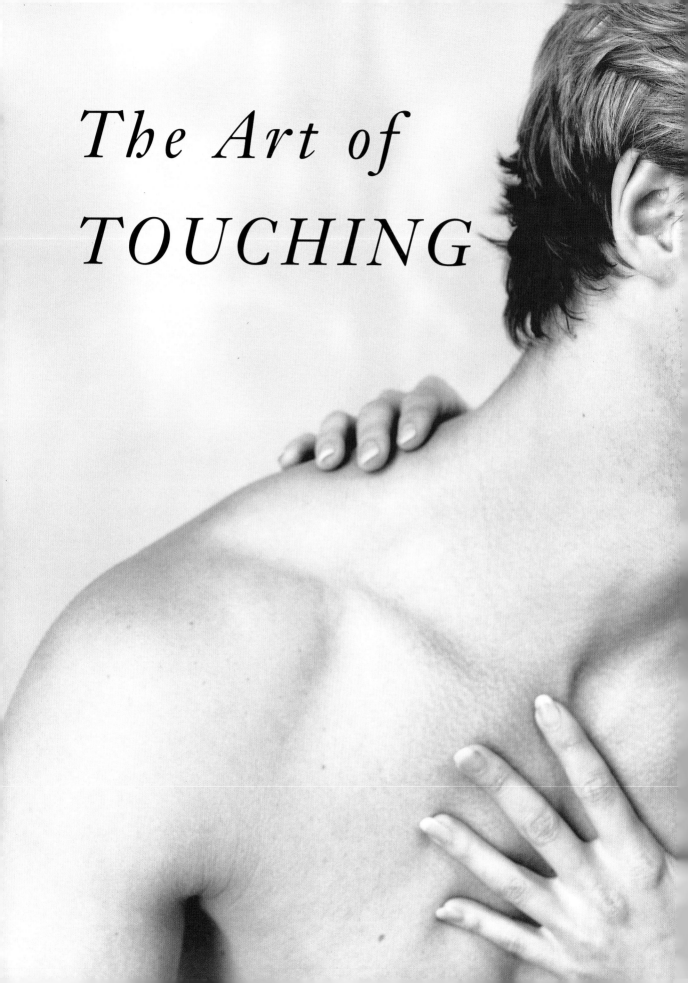

The Art of
TOUCHING

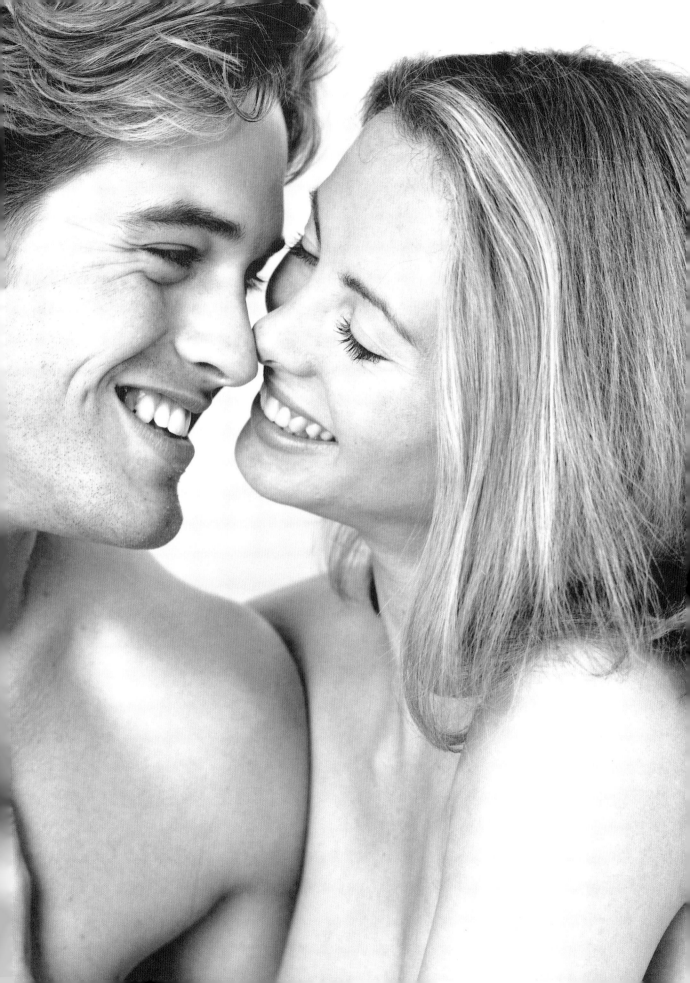

TECHNIQUES

Massage is about touch, and touch is communication. Thoughts and feelings can be communicated through our hands. How we touch can reflect and alter our partner's feelings and our own, which flow back and forth as our partner responds. The quality of our touch can transform a massage into a beautifully evocative, creative experience.

However, no matter how gentle a person's feelings are for their partner, massage involves structured touch, which must be learnt to be accomplished properly. The three basic types of touch, which are used regularly in this book, are effleurage, petrissage and friction.

Effleurage is an oiling stroke, good for getting to know your partner's body. Petrissage uses a pumping, kneading motion, which is wonderful for releasing tension. Friction presses into specific problems, and, best used for small areas, gives a feeling of deep release.

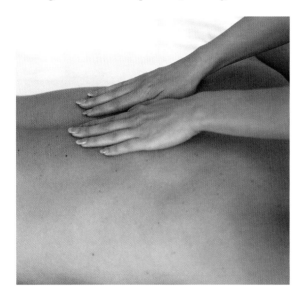

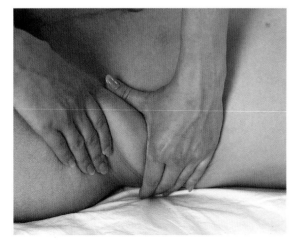

effleurage

This is the first stroke of any massage, and is used to spread the oil, as well as to make contact and explore your partner's body. Starting with your hands flat, fingers relaxed, glide lightly down the body, feeling for knots or tension (top left). Allow your fingers to spread as you sweep round to return, gradually trailing off with the fingertips. Generally, you should increase the pressure as you stroke towards the heart. This stroke relaxes, affecting the nerves beneath the skin, and helps return the blood flow to the heart.

petrissage

Here deeper strokes, good for fleshy areas, are used. Kneading is the most useful example. Grasp the flesh, pushing your thumb in and away from you. Use your fingers to roll the flesh back towards you (bottom left). Like kneading dough, move your hands alternately, with a squeezing, rolling, lifting action. Kneading frees the muscle fibers, increasing circulation.

friction

Here, the thumbs are used to apply specific pressure to joints, deep tissue and muscle over bone. Press down using the pad of your thumb, circling slightly on the spot for penetration (main picture). Friction brings release and stimulates circulation.

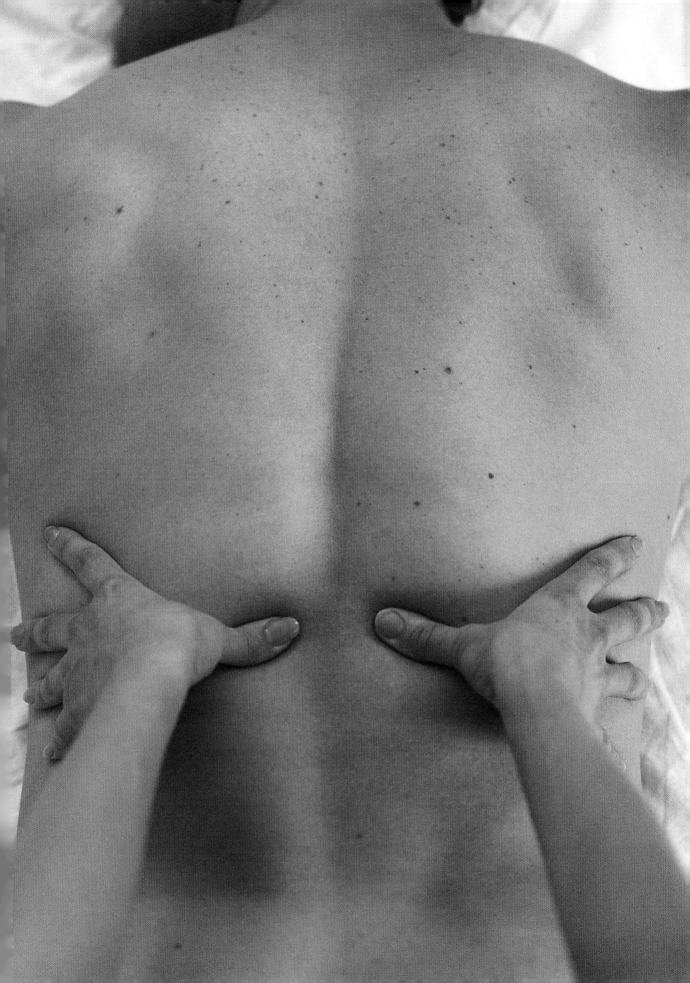

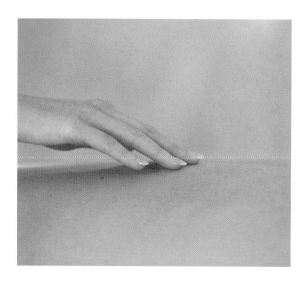

fingertips

The surface of the skin contains billions of nerve endings stimulated by the lightest touch. Using featherlight strokes you can increase its sensitivity. Using the pads of your fingers, lightly trail down your partner's skin. 'Walk' your fingers down his back for light sensations. Gently caress the delicate areas of his face and run your fingers through his hair. When stroking with your fingers, keep your wrists relaxed and flexible and break any contact gently. Brush strokes will make the transition softly from one area of the body to another.

flat of hand

The flat of the hand can be used for introductory strokes and to 'iron out' across the back, moving outwards from beside the spine. The movement can also be used where stronger pressure is needed, for example, along the thigh. The flat of the hand used softly gives a warm sense of

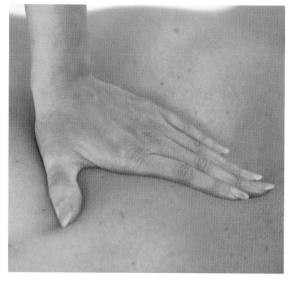

contact. You can use it to circle, or put one hand on top of the other, increasing the pressure in the center. For a slight variation, you can also tilt your hand, increasing the pressure either at the edge or the forefinger joint. This is useful when working round the shoulder blade.

rolling thumbs

As well as using the pads of the thumbs to press, the thumbs can also be used in a rolling movement. Tilting your thumbs very slightly, use the whole length of your thumb to push the muscle away from you. In a rolling movement, one thumb continues where the other stopped. Keep the rolls reasonably short, and by using your thumbs alternately, you create a feeling of one continuous flow. Rolling can be used to work down alongside the spine, on the soles of the feet, palms, or gently down the nose. The fingers can be curled or spread, but press only with the thumbs.

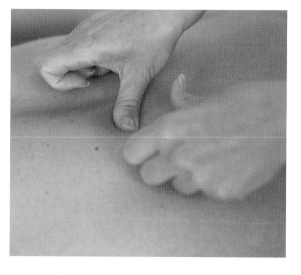

knuckles

Curl your fingers into a fist, with your thumb tucked in or protruding and bend your wrist over so your knuckles are exposed. Now press down into the flesh, using a circling, twisting motion, being attentive to your partner's pressure needs. The knuckles are only used for fleshy, resistant areas, particularly the buttocks and, with care, the soles of the feet. By rippling your fingers as you 'knuckle', an intriguing sensation is produced, altering the intensity of the pressure. Keep your wrist straight while knuckling, as this gives strength to the movement.

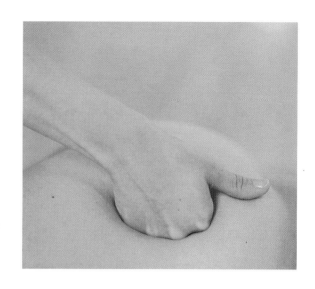

heel

Bend your wrist back, lift your palm and fingers slightly and push away from you, along the muscle, with the heel. This gives the stroke added strength, penetrates the muscle deeply, and gives a satisfying sensation. The heel can be used where added strength is needed, such as the thigh muscles. It is used for deep circling, especially over firm, fleshy areas, like the buttocks. It can be used to probe and press into muscular areas, while not losing any sensitivity from your touch. Keep your elbow slightly bent to create an angle between your shoulder, elbow and wrist.

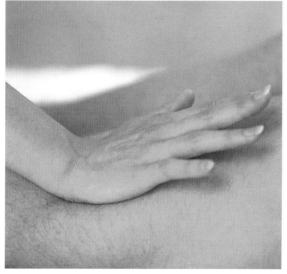

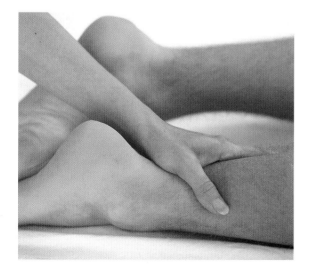

tiger's mouth

So called to describe the shape of the hands when the thumb and forefinger are spread, this position, also known as a 'V', is used to squeeze along muscles after effleurage. Place your thumb and forefinger on either side, adjusting the angle to comfortably fit around the muscles. Push upwards, away from you, adjusting the angle of your hand to accommodate the muscles' increased bulk. Push as far as you can with a firm pressure, but not too hard, until you reach along the muscles' length. You may prefer to use both hands, one behind the other, to give the movement extra strength.

THE ART OF TOUCHING – techniques

23

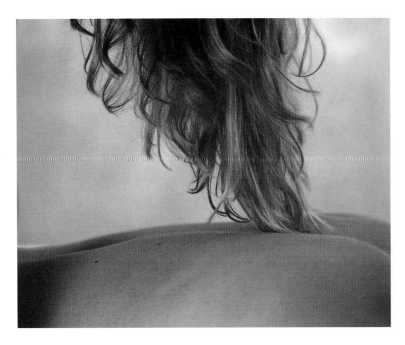

be creative

In sensual massage, you can be creative with your body, both in keeping contact with your partner and the parts you use to touch. Hair feels particularly good on the body, either sweeping over the skin, or small flicks over hands and feet. Full body brushes, with skin touching or tantalizingly close, arouse exciting sensations. As you massage, use all parts of your body for contact, arousing your partner's senses and increasing pleasure for you.

Within the range of traditional movements (see page 20), there is a whole world of versatility, literally at your fingertips. For large sweeping movements, being precise, or simply for different sensations, every part of the hand can work to subtle effect. Different parts of the hand can be used to increase pressure, to touch lightly or playfully tease. Try these variations out on your partner, increasing confidence and ability as you experiment. As you massage, do not limit your movements to your hands. By using your whole body you can increase pleasure in imaginative ways.

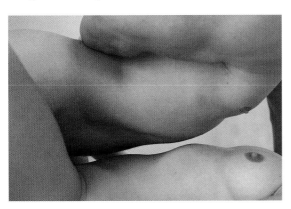

Keep the body contact close and sensitive, using rubs and brushes for sensation and delight. A whole body brush is a wonderful experience, while trailing, especially flicking, hair has a pleasurably unexpected feel.

We all instinctively have different ways to touch that convey different messages. Whether we are feeling loving, relaxed, sensual, or playful – we spontaneously express ourselves. The parts of our bodies that we use to express the tenderness of love can be very different from, say, erotic arousal. In a loving massage, we make use of these different nuances, when senses and receptivity are heightened. Like rolling waves, sensual caresses follow strokes for deep relaxation. Erotic arousal becomes dispersed through playful teasing, constantly affirming feelings of love. Sensual massage is a gift of your 100 per cent concentration, an experience to which your partner need only respond. It is an intimate way of expressing your feelings about each other. Like a unique conversation, each massage will be different.

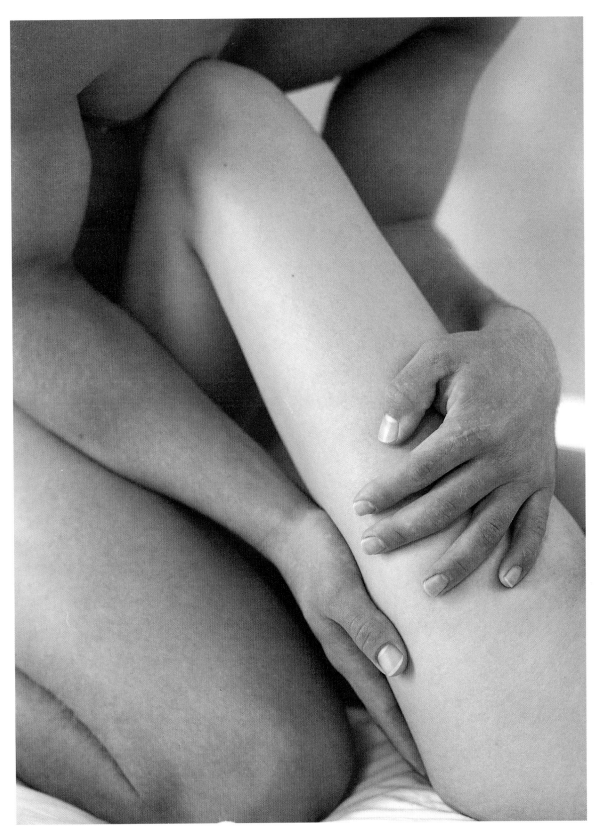

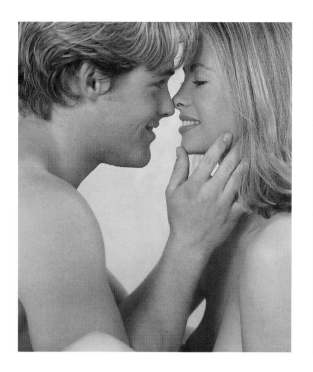

the loving touch _This expresses the tenderness and closeness we feel, the softness the other arouses in us._

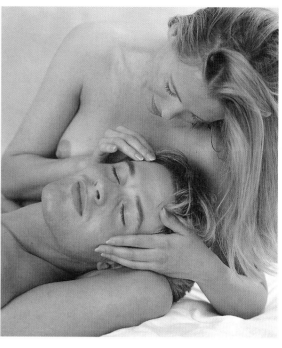

the relaxing touch _Calm and soothing, we comfort and relieve strain softly with gentle strokes._

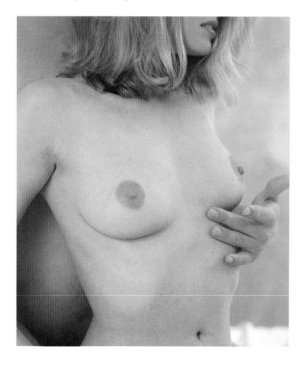

the erotic touch _Use this to arouse your lover, stimulating both the body and sexual fantasy._

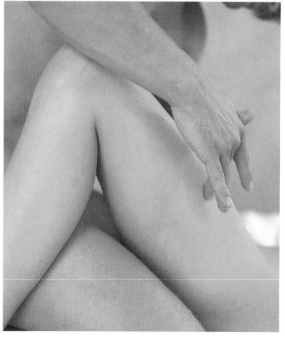

the sensual touch _The experience of feeling our partner through our skin and giving great pleasure._

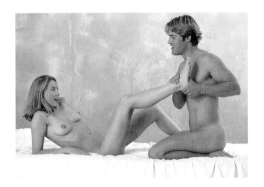

the stimulating touch *This can come as a surprise, waking and alerting your partner. An invigorating touch, it sends pulses throughout the body. Good for sharpening the senses, it gives an immediate energy lift.*

the playful touch *For fun, to make each other laugh, to play together and to let go together. Teasing each other soon gets rid of seriousness and is a great tension release and natural restorer. Use the ways you naturally touch your partner in addition to your massage strokes. Above all, bring a sense of playfulness to the massage, so that it remains an enjoyable experience. As you approach the massage in an adventurous spirit, a sense of fun will be a vital ingredient. Experiment with touching each other and totally give in to pleasure.*

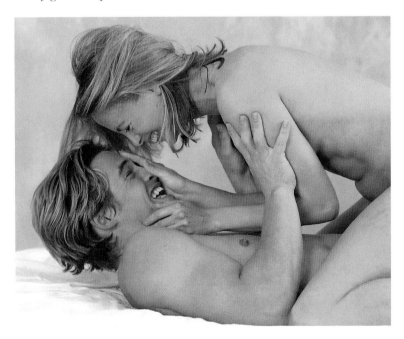

Massage for
RELAXATION

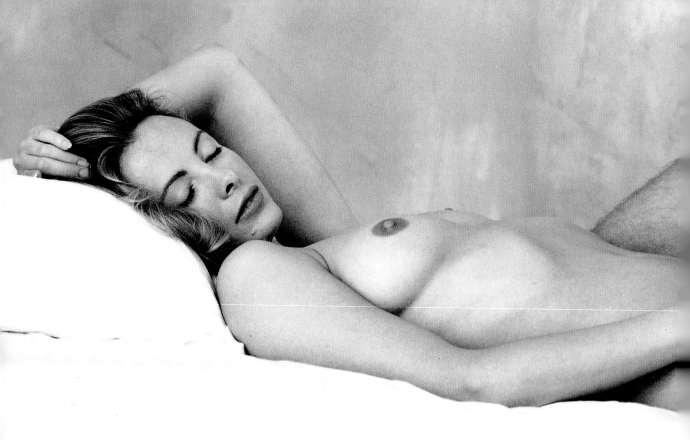

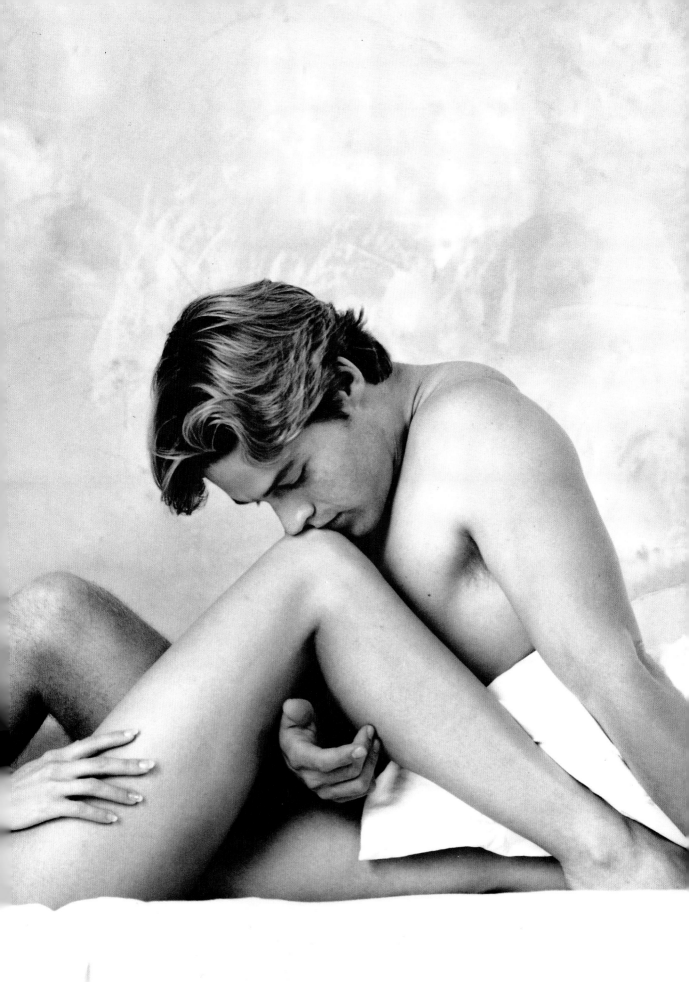

A RELAXATION MASSAGE

Make sure, first of all, you are happy to give a massage, then check the room for lighting and warmth. Do the relaxation exercises (see pages 14-17) to prepare yourself, tuning in to your own body and how you feel. Make sure you have some oil prepared, that the answering machine is on, and you have enough room so as not to feel restricted.

When giving a massage, especially if it is new to you, it is important to sit and move correctly from the start. Sit on your

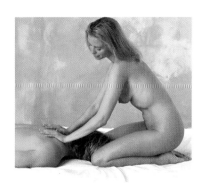

1. easing tension

To begin the massage, kneel at your partner's head, lean forwards and gently rest your hands on his shoulders (above right). Simply feel the contact. Imagine the flow of energy from you to your partner. At this point, your hands may

pick up information about how your partner is feeling, how tense or relaxed he is. Noting anything you feel, make this a moment simply to connect. After oiling your hands, glide gently down the back (below left), as if your hands were molded to your

partner's body. Spread your hands at the lower back (below center) and sweep upwards to the shoulders in one long continuous movement (below). Repeat several times to ease tension, ending the strokes flowing down the arms. This is a gentle introductory movement.

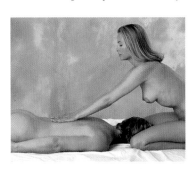
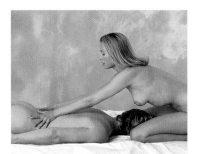
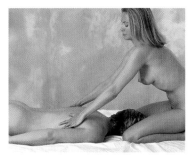

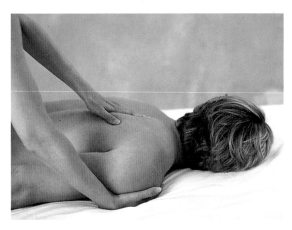

2. knead, squeeze and roll

Move to the side and place one hand under your partner's shoulder, and one hand on top, close to his shoulder blade. Gently ease the muscles round the blade, at the same time as pulling slightly toward you with the lower hand (left). Use a gentle kneading movement along the top of the shoulder, starting at the outer edge and moving towards the neck (right). Squeeze and roll to ease any tension, taking care not to dig in too deep. When you reach the neck, return, and begin again.

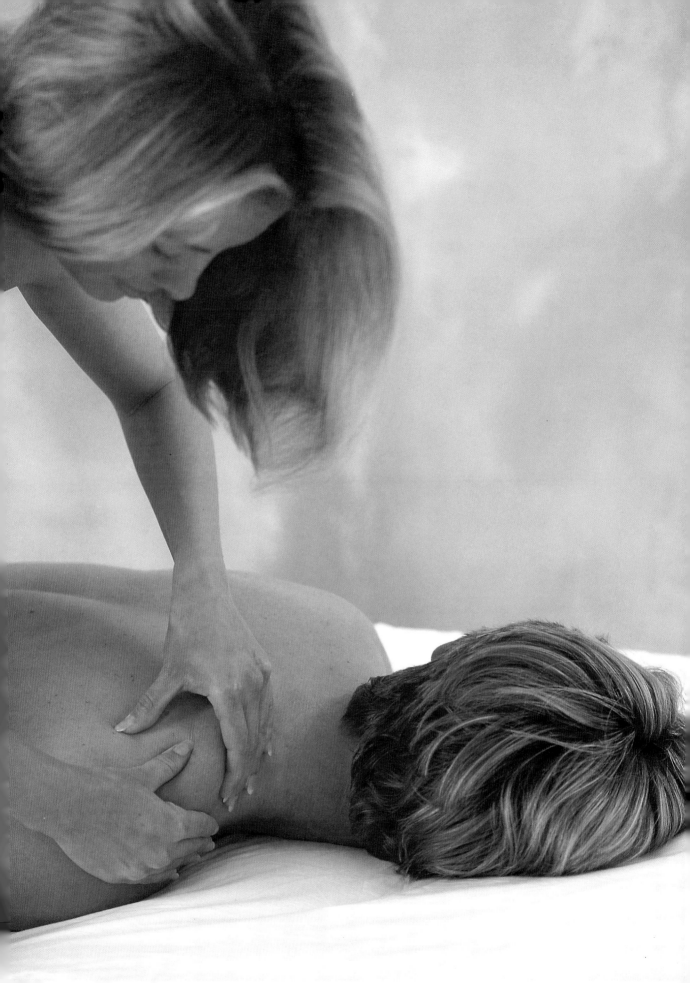

heels, have one leg up, or kneel on a cushion or pillow, but ensure that as far as is possible your spine is straight. Let the movements flow through your arms, but not come from them. Instead, involve your whole body, and move from the hips. Do not strain to exert pressure, especially if your partner is much bigger, but adjust your position and use your whole body weight. Have your hands constantly moving, except for the initial contact and final rest. Keep the flow rhythmic and continuous.

Listen to your partner's body, being aware of the way it changes, and see how it reacts to your strokes. From the beginning, check with your partner for pressure, encouraging feedback on what feels good or if they want more. When receiving massage, thoughts and emotions come and go, flitting like clouds across the sky. Be receptive if your partner wants to share these impressions with you, or respect their need for quietness and space.

THE BENEFITS OF A RELAXATION MASSAGE
In a natural state of health, we deal with stress and tension. After tensing up, we would then let go. In a sedentary, restricted lifestyle, with

3. rolling thumbs

Now return to your partner's head, and using the movement of rolling thumbs, work the triangle between the base of your partner's neck and the shoulder. Beginning in the angle where you finished the kneading movement, push down, rolling diagonally toward the spine. Do this movement several times, stopping an inch short of the spine.

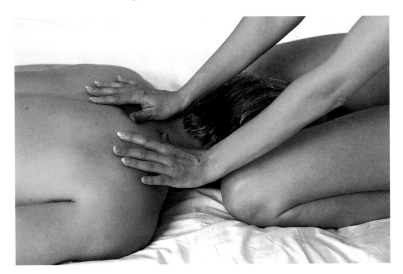

4. rolling down the spine

This movement is a continuation, and brings the thumbs down the length of the spine. Increase the length of the rolls, keeping an inch away from the spine, and using alternating strokes down to the lower back. Then, before reaching the pelvic bone return to the upper back and repeat the movement a number of times. This flowing, rhythmic rolling disperses tension.

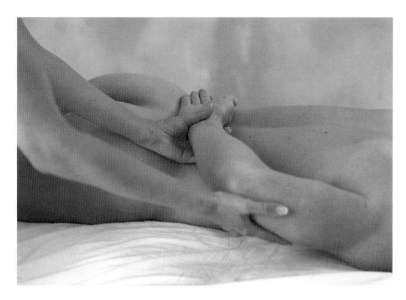

5. shoulder and arm

Move to your partner's side and pick up the arm, supporting the wrist and elbow (left). Place the arm behind your partner's back, so the shoulder blade is exposed. Supporting the shoulder with one hand underneath, with the other, work round the shoulder blade (below, left). Using the flat of your hand to follow the contour, begin at the top of the shoulder and pull

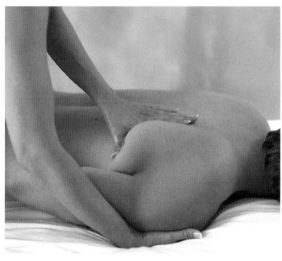

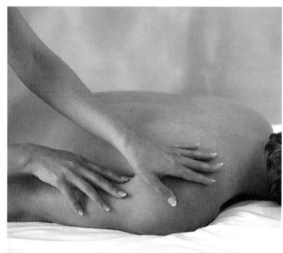

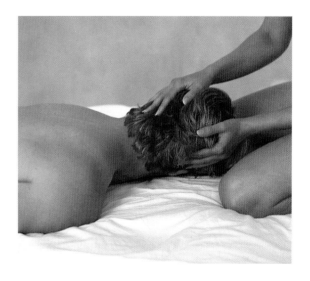

round. Work right round to the shoulder joint, and after completing the stroke several times, slide down to the hand. Pick up the arm, again supporting the wrist and elbow, and return the arm gently to your partner's side. Starting at the shoulder, use very light brushstrokes to trickle down the arm to the fingertips (above right). In a movement like a waterfall, repeat this many times. The stroke, while light and sensitive, should be quite defined. Kneel at your partner's head and ask him to slowly turn it, using your hands gently as a guide. With the head turned (right), you are ready to repeat the movements on the other shoulder.

increasing demands and pressure, the tendency is for the stress to build up. This has a negative effect on us. We become neurotic, agitated, anxious, our minds constantly overactive and unable to switch off. Sleeping or eating badly, using drugs or alcohol, we lose touch with ourselves and damage our relationships. Physically, we become tense, our muscles can harden and tighten; we may suffer from headaches, back problems and restricted movement.

The beauty of massage is that it is a natural treatment, it feels good and can have a profound effect on us. Massaging the muscles frees up any congestion. Loosening contracted muscle fibers, it aids the elimination of waste products via the blood and lymph. Massage stimulates the circulation, can lower blood pressure, and has a tonic effect on the nerves. The nerves relate directly to our organs, so it is often the case that massage can regulate the body, helping it function more efficiently. The energy that was diverted to maintaining a state of tension is now released, and the feeling is more vibrant. Through the effect on the nervous system, the mind can gradually quieten, producing an all-over feeling of well-being.

6. effleuraging the buttocks

After massaging the upper back, move down your partner's body to effleurage the buttocks. Put a little oil on your hands, then place them on the top to begin the stroke. With a gliding movement, hands molded to the body, sweep out and round, following the contour of the hips. Keep the movement generous, and following the swell of flesh, come round to the crease and sweep upwards to start again. This movement focuses sensation on the buttocks, in preparation for the deeper strokes to follow. At the same time as being extremely pleasurable to massage, the buttocks can carry a lot of tension, which is not actually felt. So use your hands to sense out your partner's muscles, and, if tense, they should begin to release under your hands. The buttocks contain the strong gluteal muscles, so the pressure you use in this area can be reasonably firm. Remember to start with your hands in a sort of diving position, then spread the fingers to include as much flesh as you can. As many people spend much of their lives sitting down, this particular movement can give enormous satisfaction.

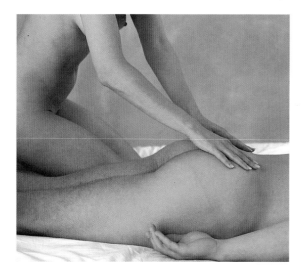
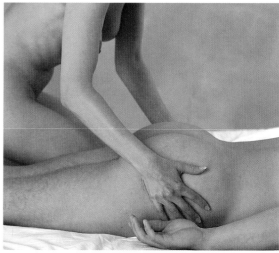

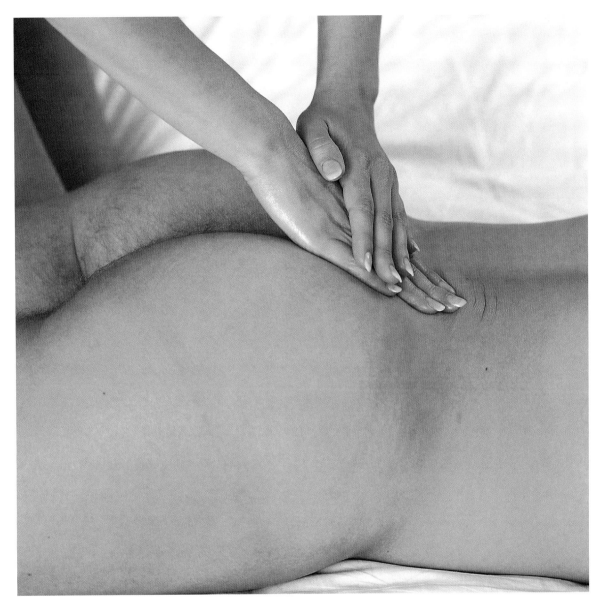

7. circling the sacrum

Placing one hand on top of the other for a steady pressure, position your hands over your partner's sacrum. This is the central, bony triangle that ends just below where the buttock crease begins. With the movement going anti-clockwise, circle your hands broadly around the sacrum's shape. Keep your fingers flat over the bone, applying a steady, medium-light pressure. This stroke dispels a lot of tension. In the sacral area lies an important nerve center, mainly connecting to the legs. By easing in this way the nerves are soothed, and your partner will feel the effect in the legs, hips and lower back. Check to make sure the pressure feels right and that you are not applying fingertip pressure as you move. The circling should be slow, generous, and feel extremely satisfying, both to the one receiving and the one who gives. After completing the circles several times, you will feel loosening in the area as a whole. This signals it is now time to turn your attention back to the buttocks.

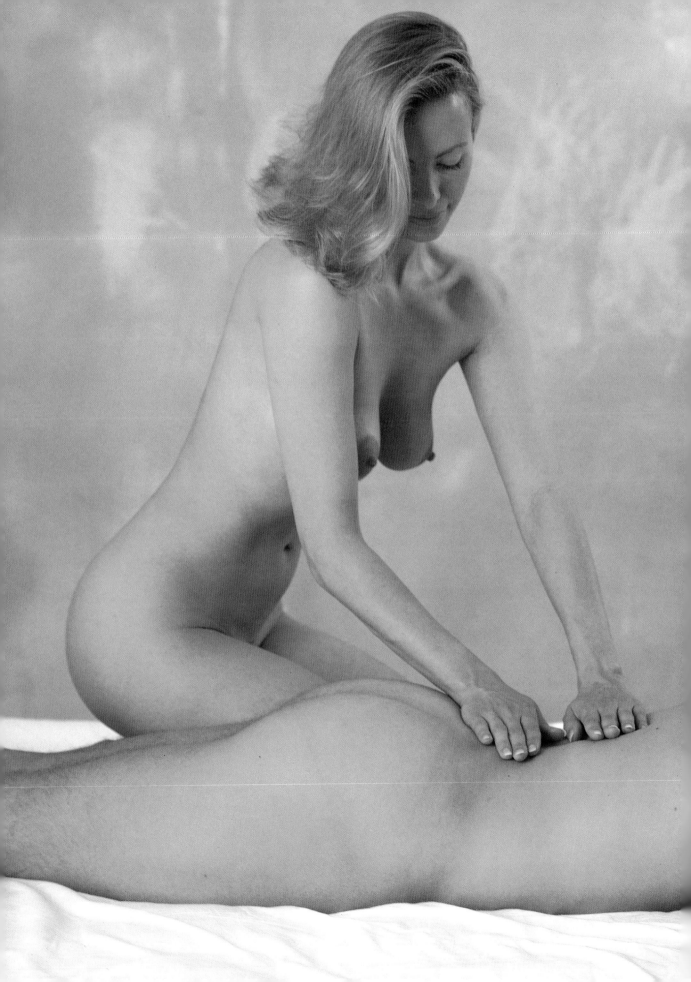

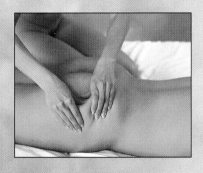

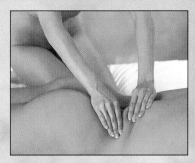

particular attention between the shoulder blades, and from there, hop down the rest of the spine, still with the thumbs. This should be quite light and bouncy, pressing briefly, at larger intervals, down to the lower back (below). From here,

8. kneading the back

Leaning across to your partner's opposite buttock, begin to knead, rolling and squeezing the flesh (above). Firm, lively pressure feels good here; the movement should be deep and liberating. The kneading movement continues naturally up the back (above right), following the spine, an inch away, right up to the neck. Although the movement here will be narrower and more shallow, the effect is wonderfully far-reaching. Switch

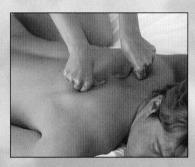

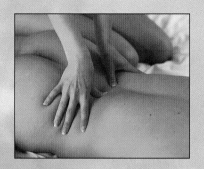

sides, and repeat these two movements, then come down the back, using your thumbs (above). Press with the pads, at even intervals, into the muscle bands either side of the spine. Pay

trail your fingers down the lower spine, then place your hands to rest across the back (main picture). Spend some moments here, just both of you resting. It is a soft and gentle way to complete the back.

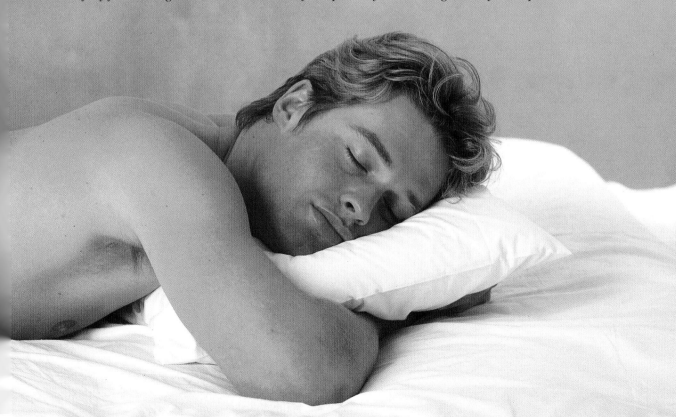

The Joy of Giving

Perhaps the real heart of massage is the human contact that it provides. Just being touched and affirmed is often enough. When giving massage, take care not to be judge-mental; it is a process of coming together, not one of standing back. Through massage we once again feel comfortable with our bodies, rediscovering just how great the body feels. Feeling new, we see the world with fresh eyes, rediscovering our enthusiasm for simple things.

As the person giving massage, we can do a lot for our partner. It is a wonderful skill to develop. Giving is also relaxing, so as we

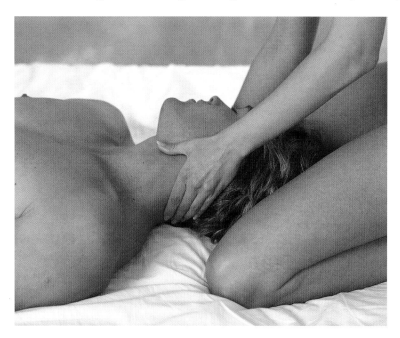

9. rolling the head

Apply a little oil to your hands. With your partner on his back, neck straight, place your hands on either side of the head. Cup your hands around the base, fingers touching at the back of the neck. Now, roll your partner's head using your left hand, the right hand giving light support. The head should roll quite naturally. If your partner is tense, encourage him to let go. Repeat using your right hand, and gently roll the head the other way.

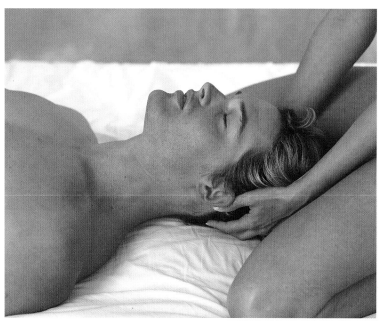

10. pulling the neck

Place your hands under the neck, cupping around the base of the head. Pull back gently toward you, keeping your fingers under the bony ridge of the skull. The direction of the pull is like a continuation of the spine, pulling back, rather than up. Do this movement just once.

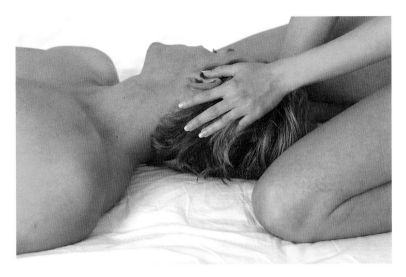

11. turning the head

To turn the head, cup both hands on either side, your thumbs in front of the ears, forefingers behind. Now, cradling the head, turn it very gently, so it rests on top of your hand. The beauty of receiving massage is that, for once, there is no need to make an effort of any kind.

12. pushing the shoulder

With your right hand still supporting the head, slide your left down your partner's neck and along the shoulder. When you reach the edge of the shoulder, gently push down away from you, giving the neck muscles a satisfying stretch. To increase the stretch, pull slightly with your right hand. Again, you should do this movement just one time.

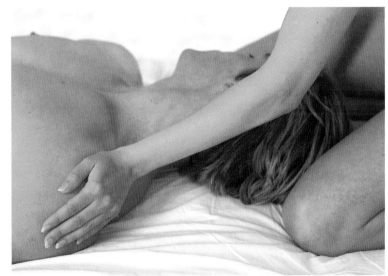

13. rotating the scalp

Return your left hand to your partner's head, and spreading your fingers, press down with the pads. Now use your whole hand to make a circling movement on the scalp, feeling skin move over bone. Rotate one area, then move on. Turn your partner's head to repeat movements 12 and 13.

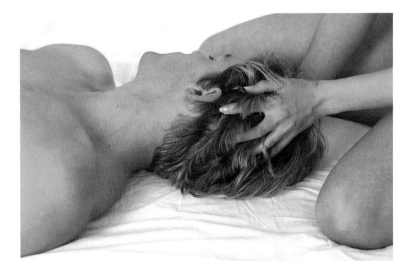

massage, our own bodies also let go. In being the giver, you are the one taking responsibility for a while, so it is up to you to make sure you have everything you will need.

A relaxation massage is a completely different experience. You will find out many new things about your partner. Getting to know your partner's tension means knowing your partner better. To relieve that tension is an invaluable gift. The massage is for your enjoyment, so as you both relax, the pleasure will flow between you.

We all experience the need to relax, to have time when there are no demands put upon us. To have the luxury of regaining our equilibrium, letting stresses and strains simply drain away. Through a relaxation massage, the process of relaxing and being relaxed by our partner creates a special atmosphere of intimacy and trust. Putting ourselves, literally, into our partner's hands increases the understanding on both sides. At the same time, being refreshed and in a relaxed frame of mind leads on to greater creativity, and in turn, to better sex. When giving a relaxation massage, your mind is on your partner, and your wish and ability to help. While sensually pleasurable, the massage relaxes rather than arouses. There is no pressure on your partner to respond. Satisfaction comes as your partner visibly lets go, a smile of enjoyment and relief creeping across his or her face.

If the relaxation massage is to be successful, your partner must want to relax. It is no good going through the motions with someone who is unwilling to receive. It is a decision taken before you start, and is your partner's most important contribution to the massage.

14. completing the relaxation massage
Having completed work on the scalp and neck, press with thumbs together up your partner's forehead. Move in a straight line from between the eyebrows, pressing gently with your thumb pads, towards the hairline. Continue the movement through the hair to the center of the head. This movement, while releasing forehead tension, can be felt easing tightness in the jaw. Resting, with your hands cupping the head, completes the massage.

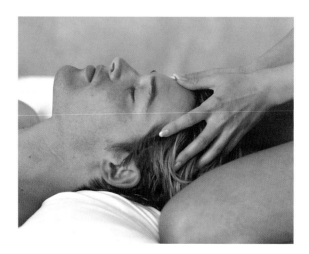

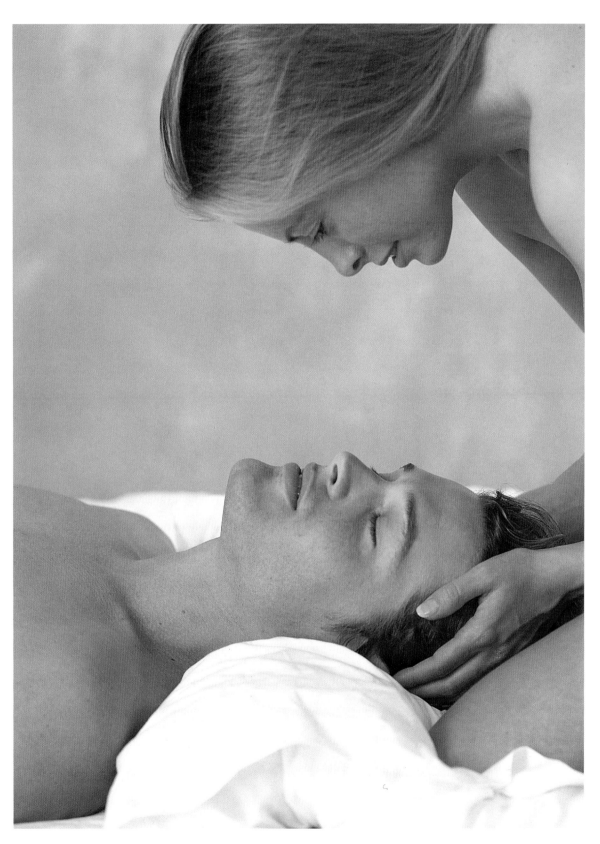

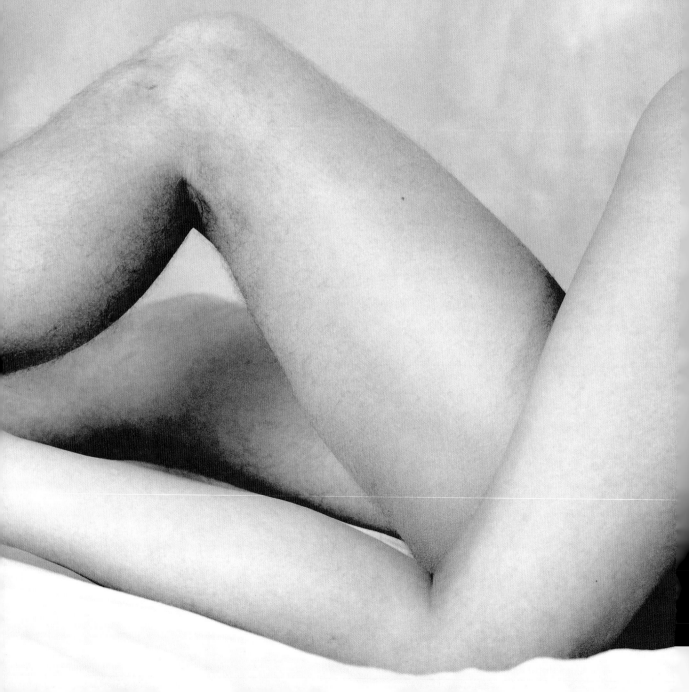

A Full Sensual
MASSAGE

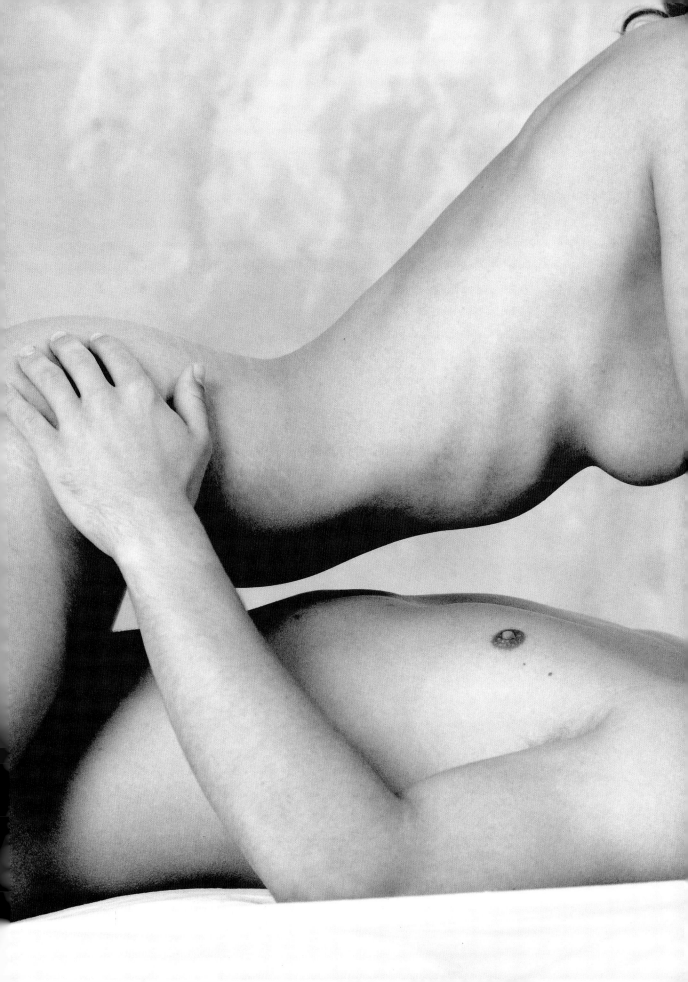

THE SENSUAL TOUCH

Giving your partner a full sensual body massage is almost an extension of the movements with which you will now be familiar. A sensual massage incorporates the strokes used for relaxation with caresses to arouse and stimulate. While you relax your partner's body, you arouse and heighten the senses through your movements. As you use your hands, your fingertips play over your partner, making contact, releasing slowly, and promising more. Allow the movements of the massage to draw your partner's senses to your hands as they move in gentle, flowing erotic rhythms.

The quality of your touch, the way you use your hands, changes when you give a sensual massage. It is a powerful combination. Soft, releasing strokes, firm pressure strokes to penetrate the muscles, together with light, tantalizing

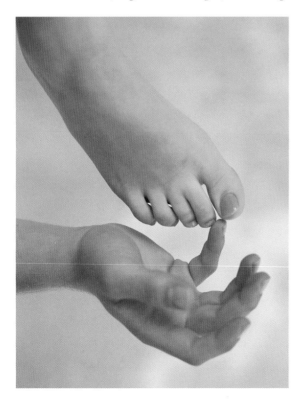

touches. The changes go in cycles, the movements rhythmic and flowing, blending from one into the next. To relax your partner use soft, soothing strokes to explore the body and ease away any immediate tension. The pressure, while gentle, is definite and firm. Deep pressure strokes go right into the body, reducing any build-up of tension in the muscles. The relief of being touched so deeply is almost tangible. To enhance your sensual strokes, use a lighter touch that is less defined, releasing slowly, and lingering as you finish. For example, after squeezing up a muscle, gently release your hand, then trail your fingers delicately along the skin. The final moments of the movement become almost imperceptible. As you massage, use your hands to build the excitement for your partner, then through stillness discharge the feelings you have aroused throughout the body.

When you give a massage for relaxation, your body movements are unobtrusive, the focus being the therapeutic benefits for your partner. As you give a sensual massage, try to involve your body more and your enjoyment and wholeheartedness will be communicated to your partner. Sensual brushes and full skin contact will enhance your partner's experience, adding to the sensual pleasure. During massage, pay attention to the nuances of touch, exploring and making contact creatively. Every stroke should be a source of pleasure for your partner, so it is important to listen to the reponses of the body. You will very quickly feel or sense if something is not quite right. Ask your partner to provide feedback as you go along. Far from detracting from the massage this enhances your communication. The beauty comes when you are so fine-

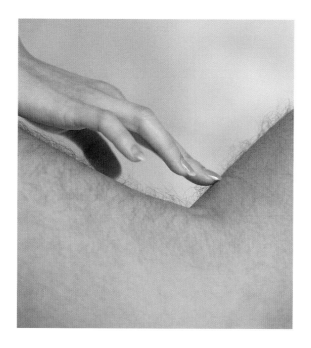

ly tuned to each other that needs and responses are completely automatic. At first you will need to practice a little. While the hands learn surprisingly fast, the most important factor is the flow of feelings from your heart. If you are massaging simply to give to your partner, your partner's body will trust your hands. Trust is a vital ingredient of the massage and increases as the experience progresses. The massage should be an affirmation of your partner. As you will discover, there is nothing so deeply erotic. As you perform the movements, use the sounds of your breathing, your own unique noises, to please and arouse your partner. There can be nothing more enjoyable for your partner than to know that you are receiving pleasure from giving massage. This applies equally as you receive. Express your appreciation and satisfaction.

Through sensual massage, each area of the body is brought to life, in a process of continuing discovery. The soft, inner parts of the body are extremely sensual and erotic. For example, the crook of the elbow, the throat or the back of the knee will all tingle with sensuality when touched. While special areas of the body stimulate more than others, arousing massage makes the whole body an erogenous zone. Take time to touch and explore, deriving pleasure from each new discovery. Use the process of the massage to create and be inventive, developing the eroticism of the body. Touching sensually and sensitively, you can electrify your partner increasing the intensity between you.

In the following pages you have a step-by-step guide to a full, flowing sensual massage. Each stage and movement follows on from the next, covering both the back and the front of the body. The movements from the relaxation massage are also included. Use the sequence to guide you, incorporating your own experience and ideas, and of course your own unique knowledge of your partner. Also included is more general information to give you further insights into the body and more especially into your partner. Everything is there simply to be used. Enjoy bringing the strokes to life.

THE BACK

The back is a wonderful area to massage. Rich with nerves and powerful muscles, more than any other area, it cries out to be touched. In good health our backs supply us with energy, are a source of protection, suppleness and strength. Very much a source of sensual pleasure, the back affects the way we walk, the way we move, hold ourselves and sit. By massaging the back the whole body is affected, renewing that vital connection with ourselves. Massaging the back is an extremely effective way to begin the full sensual massage. Once it is relaxed and aroused, the whole body responds.

PREPARING FOR THE MASSAGE

With a sensual massage, just as with a relaxation massage, the important opening steps set the tone for everything that follows. The first contact speaks volumes. Be totally receptive to your partner, her mood, stillness or inner vibrancy. Sense the feelings of anticipation increase. Be totally willing to give. At the same

1. effleuraging the back

Before you begin the massage, kneel at your partner's head (above) and gently stroke the hair away from her face. Rest your fingers softly on the back of the head and neck before beginning the massage. Let your fingertips sense your partner, at the same time as your own feelings begin to flow out through your hands. Apply a little oil to your hands, then begin to effleurage your partner's back (near right). As you sweep down the back, be aware of the muscle curves, the color and texture of the skin. Allow your hands to fan and undulate over your partner's body, applying only very light pressure as you pass over its contours. Glide down toward your partner's lower back (main picture), moving over the hips and buttocks with your fingertips.

Then spread your hands to come up the back once more, dragging and squeezing slightly over ribs and shoulder blades. Repeat the stroke several times to cover the entire back, easing away tension and

bringing the skin alive. As you end the movement, gently draw your hands up through your partner's hair (below), stroking through with your fingertips right to the very ends.

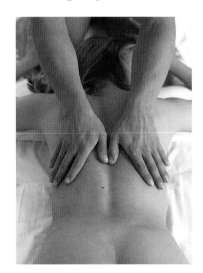

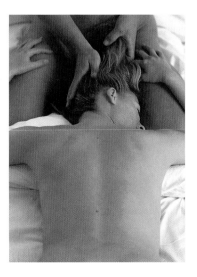

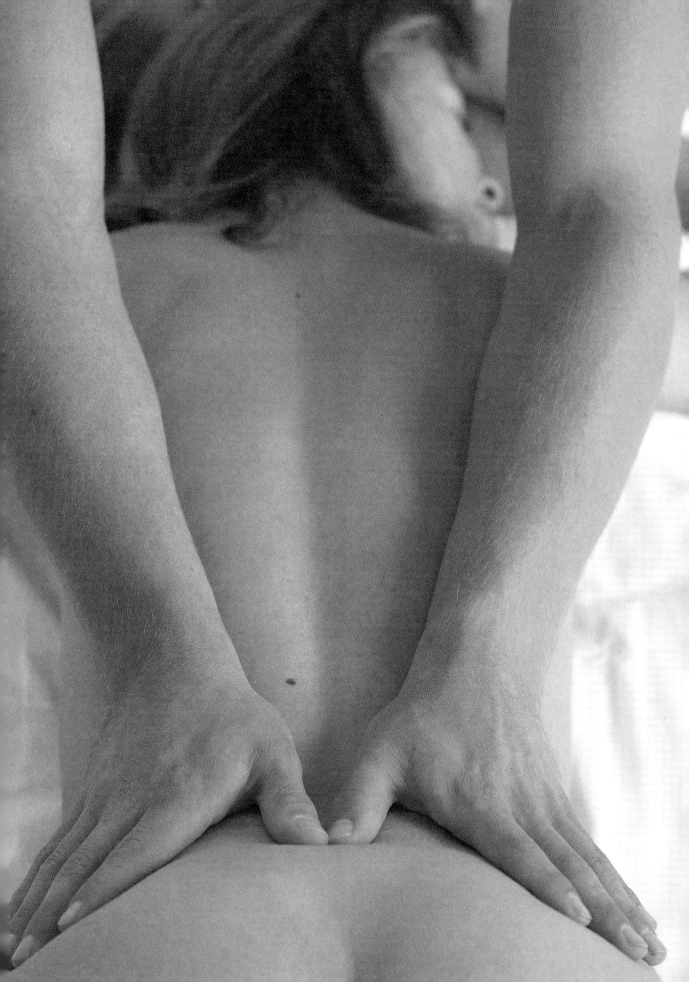

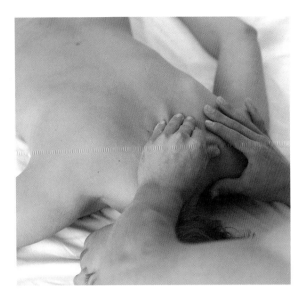 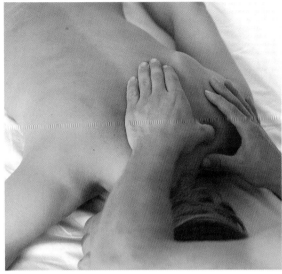

2. kneading

After you have effleuraged the whole back, you gently knead the top of the shoulder with your thumbs, squeezing the little rolls of flesh with your fingertips. Beginning at the outer edge, continue the movement to the neck, ending with longer teasing squeezes to draw your partner's senses. You should always work on the shoulder facing away from you, where the muscle is exposed. As you knead the shoulder, brush the arms or knead the neck, play with your partner's senses, varying the intensity of your touch.

3. circling

After the kneading motion, press your thumb in along the muscle, making small half-circling movements from the edge of the shoulder inwards. Press firmly to begin the circle, easing the pressure as the thumb moves round. Draw your thumb away from each circle lightly and slowly. This continues the easing effect that you began with the kneading. After easing, let the pressure trail away, continuing contact and arousal with your fingertips. Easing the muscles is much more effective than using hard pressure.

time, as your hands caress and feel out the body in the first effleurage, note the sensations your partner's skin produces in your hands. Feel the texture, any changes in roughness or smoothness, look at the color, the elasticity and the warmth. Depending on her mood, health, or the day's experience, the skin will have changed subtly from your last remembrance of it. Pay attention to your own feelings as you massage in the oil, allowing your hands to flow over the skin. Allow the invitation of your partner's skin to draw your hands into contact with the back.

GENERAL POINTS ABOUT BACK MASSAGE

The back is a large and variable area to massage and you will need to keep in mind as you work that the kind of pressure on the shoulders, lower back and buttocks needs to be different. You may find quite of a lot of tension has collected in the shoulders, especially in the 'trapezius' muscle that runs across the shoulders, neck and upper back. Pressure here should be sensitive and only slightly firm. With tight muscles it is tempting to use hard pressure but if you press too hard the muscles will fight back.

If you like, before you start the sensual massage on the shoulders, you can incorporate some of the relaxation massage (see pages 39–41). Once you have massaged the shoulders, move down to the lower back. Exploring the area, glide over the soft contours of the sacrum, buttocks and hips. The lower back can be a particularly vulnerable or strained area, and tightness here can cut off full sensations. Some relaxation movements before the sensual massage will relax the lower back and buttocks, opening your partner up to the full freedom of sensual feeling.

gentle pressure. Keeping an inch out from the spine, press evenly along the muscle bands, paying attention where you feel raised areas of muscle. Use the sensitivity of your fingers to feel the texture and tightness, and as you press correspond your movements to your partner's exhalation. As nerves branch out from the spine connecting to the whole body, this will be a highly sensitive and releasing movement for your partner. As you reach the top of the neck, bring your hands once more to your partner's lower back to draw awareness away from the

4. stroking

Move to your partner's side after completing the thumb rolls from the fleshy shoulder triangle to the spine (see page 32). Stroke down the muscles to the side of the spine with the whole of your hand, using light, caressing movements. Alternating your hands, trail lightly with your fingertips as you complete each stroke, lingering over the skin. Draw down, using these rolling brushstrokes, from the neck to the base of the spine.

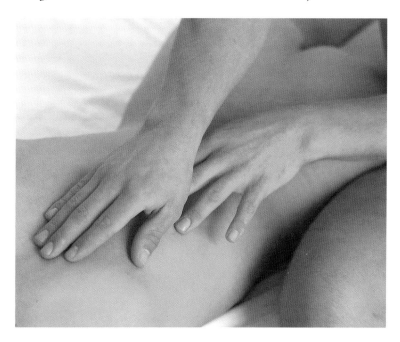

A deeper pressure used around the buttocks feels immediately satisfying and releases strong erotic, sensual feelings. Follow deep relaxation round the hips by muscle stimulation, then soft arousing skin caresses to bring the senses to life. Relaxation followed by caresses and arousal provide a combination that is difficult to resist.

When you come to massaging the spine and neck, you should be particularly careful. Both areas are very sensitive and require a more

head, and fully connect the back. This movement is also a reminder of the feelings earlier aroused, as gentle sensations diffuse throughout the body. You may choose at this point to continue the body massage, or take time to explore your partner's back in creative ways. Of all the areas of the body, the back appreciates massage most. You will find that you have to change position several times as you massage the back. Make sure you have enough room to maneuver.

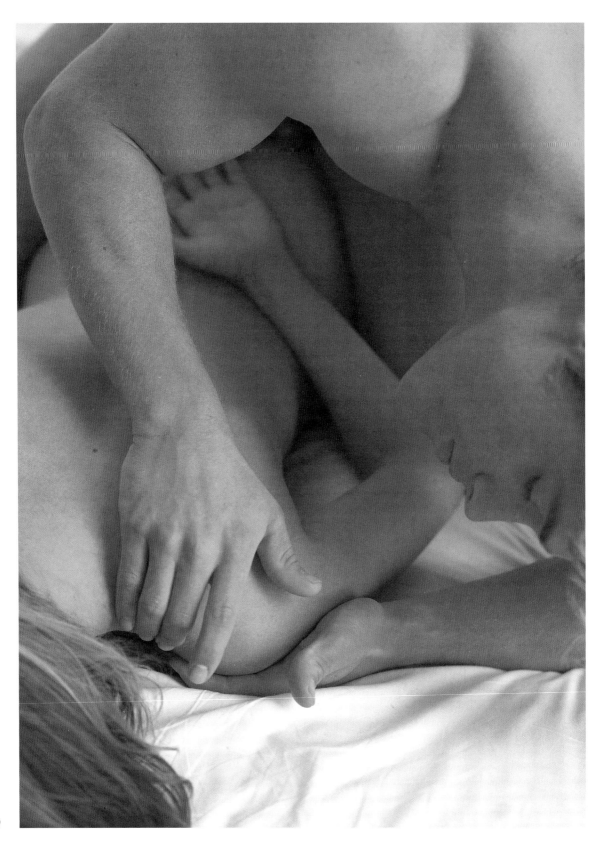

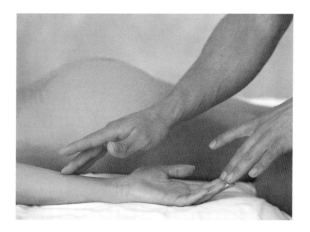

5. final strokes – kneading and brushing

To complete your massage of the upper back, move your partner's arm behind her back, easing the muscle around the shoulder blade. Still with your lower hand supporting her shoulder, use the heel of your hand to push the muscles on the blade itself (main picture). Move your hand diagonally, toward the shoulder joint, pushing slowly and deeply along the muscles. Ease the pressure to follow the contour of the shoulder down the arm. Bringing the arm back to your partner's side, use light brushstrokes all the way down to the fingertips (above). Brush slowly and sensually, until, fingertip to fingertip, you continue the sensation even after your hand has gone. Gently knead your partner's neck (below), using slow, gentle strokes to tease out any tension, then hold the hair softly as she turns her head. Knead once again, then repeat the movements on the other side.

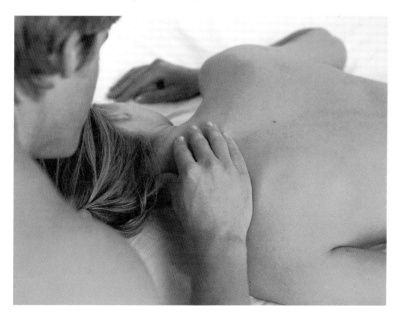

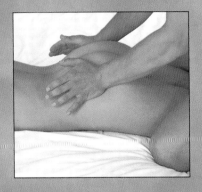
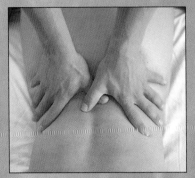

start to knead your partner's buttocks with a satisfying, generous movement. Then press in with the heel of your hand, making deep, probing, circling movements, bringing the pressure in toward you (below left). Feel the muscles, press around the hips,

6. the buttocks

Moving to your partner's legs, pour a little more oil into your hands. Now begin to effleurage the buttocks (main picture). Fan and spread your fingers, following the body contours, around the lower back, hips and the tops of the thighs. Sweep your hands upwards and outwards, shaped to the curves of flesh, until every inch is covered with a film of oil. With your hands pressing down and inwards, circle the heels into the buttocks, moving down, upwards and out to loosen the muscles (above). Try

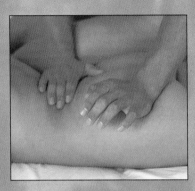
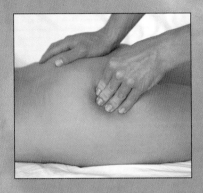

sacral circling, then spread your hands out across the back (above). As you move the hands apart, feel the dimples and the curves of the buttocks, ending the movement with your hands curved around the hips. Moving across to the side,

easing out any tensions to bring the area to life. Continue this movement with your fingertips (above), gradually easing into the hip joint to send wonderful sensations of deep release through your partner's pelvis and thighs.

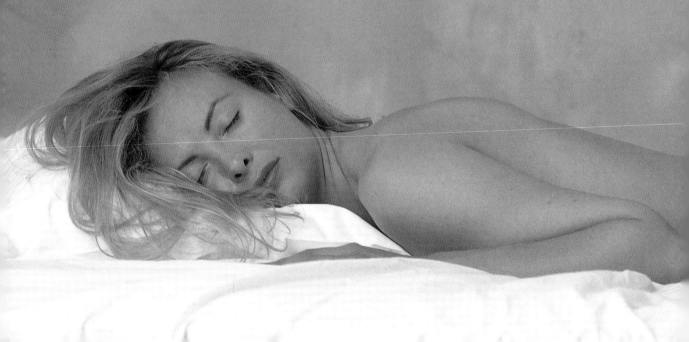

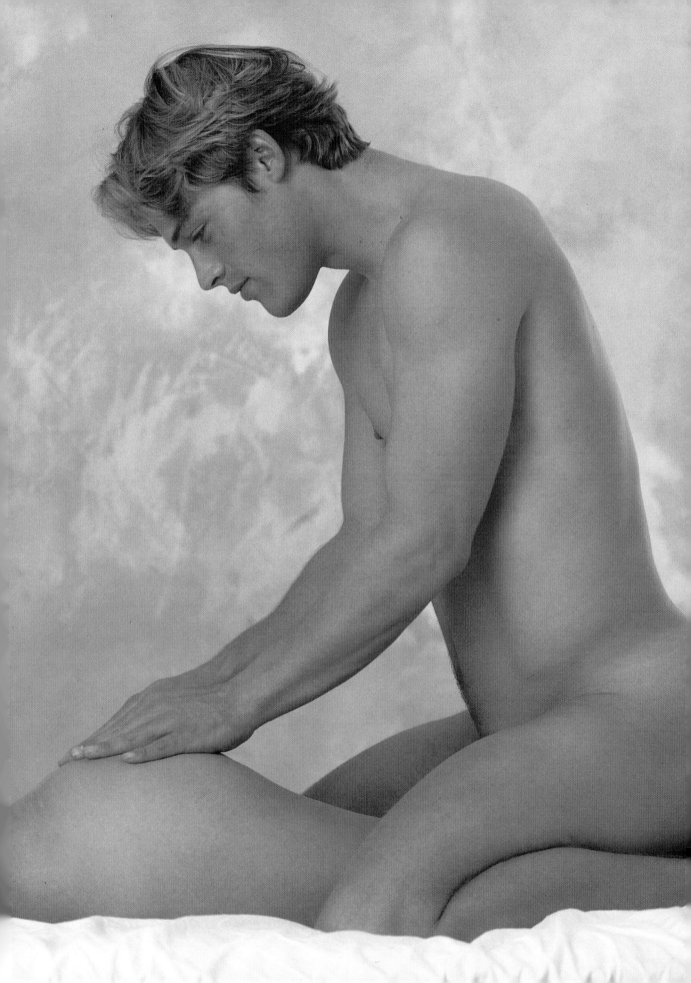

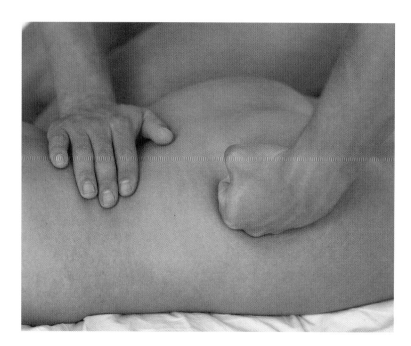

7. knuckling

To complete the deep pressure movements, form your hand into a fist, pressing firmly, yet sensitively, with your knuckles. As your hands are now familiar with the area, you will be able to loosen tension. Press into the flesh, feeling how the buttocks respond under your touch, encouraging the muscles to release and open.

BODY AWARENESS

The way we seem to see things means that we tend to divide them into parts. But the reality is that each area of the body opens into another and that every part is connected to the next. The powerful shoulders are needed for arm movement, the legs are affected by the lower back. The lower back leads into the swell of the buttocks, the ribs follow round to the swell of the breasts. Without judgement, preferences, likes or dislikes, simply open your mind as your fingers explore. With each stroke, a whole new world opens·up, every inch of skin has something different to reveal.

8. plucking

This is a light-hearted and stimulating movement that pulls the flesh away from the body. Keeping your wrists relaxed, pull mounds of flesh between your fingers and thumbs up toward you. Alternate your hands to make quick, light, plucking movements, enjoying the rippling of your partner's flesh. This playful movement will stimulate and arouse your partner, spreading tingling or tickling sensations over the buttocks and up the back.

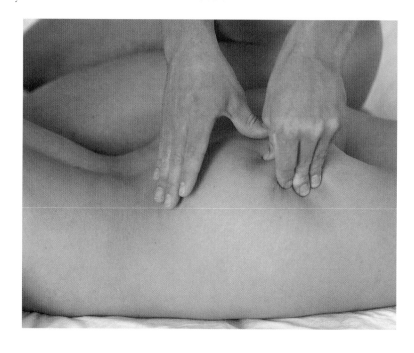

54

9. arousal

Now that the buttocks are alive and tingling, stroke up very, very lightly between them with the backs of your hands. Watch your partner's skin thrill to the touch as you continue. As sensations heighten, use a spreading stroke to diffuse erotic feelings.

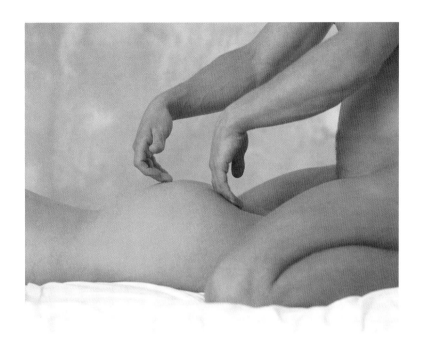

The skin is the largest organ of the body. Sensory receptors lie just below its surface, relaying messages to the central nervous system. The sense receptors responding to touch are very sensitive, and can be stimulated by extremely light pressure. Some respond to a firm pressure, while others alert the body to pain. As you massage, a lighter pressure will generally arouse and stimulate, while a heavier pressure will relax and release the body. Use variations of pressure for the sensual massage, arousing, releasing then arousing again. Let the movements and strokes blend one into the other, so alternating and changing, the rhythm remains smooth. Your partner's senses should be following your hands but left guessing, and you should not make any sudden movements.

The intimacy of the contact is very special. Profound knowledge and insights into your partner can develop. Simply keep the massage flowing, alert to your partner's response. The feelings the massage arouses in you flow through your hands, to change, rise and fall and guide your touch. As feelings increase, and your own senses are aroused, allow this to inspire your strokes. The greater your own sensations and intuitive responses, the greater your enjoyment will be. As growing enthusiasm is felt by one partner, so the other will respond in kind. Let the feelings between you build and build.

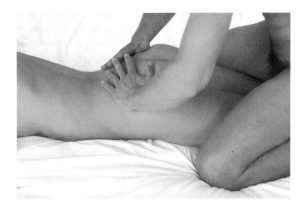

10. diffusion

Cup your hands over the sacrum, then slowly pull your hands apart, hugging them over the hips and bringing them down the thighs. Trail off with your fingertips as you complete the stroke.

55

11. 'ironing'

Move your position so that you can reach the entire back easily, in preparation for the 'ironing' stroke. Starting the movement just above the hips, position your hands either side of the spine. The heels face inwards, fingertips spreading out across the back. Then start to draw your hands apart, using a firm, even pressure, to slide your fingers around the ribs. With the whole of the flat of the hand, iron out the muscles as you push away from the spine, dispersing tension in the dorsal muscles, the broad muscles that help move the arms (right). As your heels move towards your partner's sides, add light caressing touches with your fingers to the feelings of stretch and release. Then with your fingertips, drag back toward the spine, bringing the heels of your hands back together. Position your hands for the next stroke slightly further up the back, and with no break in continuity, repeat the stroke. Work leisurely up the back. Keep the pressure on the outward strokes, your movements big and generous, which your partner will enjoy. As you come to the upper back, hook your hands around her shoulders, pulling very slightly up and back toward you (right.)

56

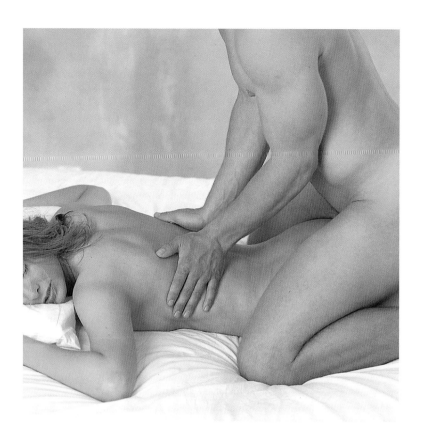

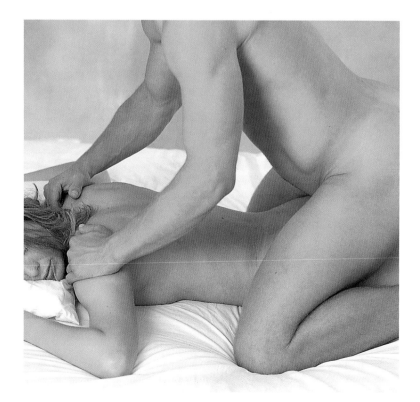

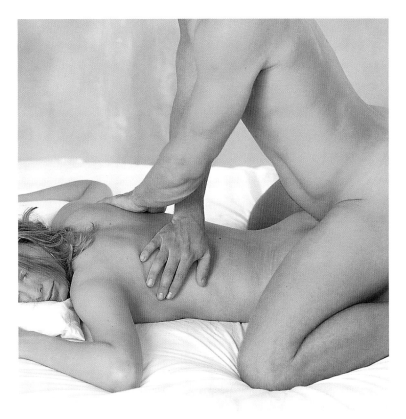

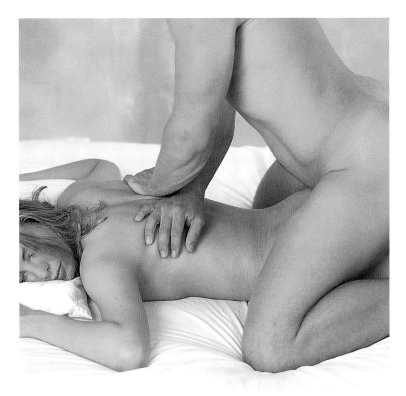

12. wringing

To continue the movement, slide your hands evenly from around the shoulders, and bring them, palms flat, towards each other. Lead with your fingers so your arms cross over each other, the hands hugging the body on opposite sides (left). Curling your fingers to the form of the body, pull your hands back toward each other, until they cross in the center of the back (below left). Continue the pressure movement as your hands slide apart from each other, moving to mold round the ribs on either side. This movement has a hugging, wringing feel, and is extremely satisfying, as first the muscles are moved in toward the spine, then slowly smoothed and stretched away. Without breaking the rhythm, use your fingertips to caress your partner's sides. As you turn your hands, point your fingers up the body. Then drag your fingers as you bring the hands back towards each other, cross over, and slide once more to the position on opposite sides. Moving slightly further down the back, repeat the wringing and returning until once again you are at the hips. Keeping the movement continuous, snaking down your partner's back, will arouse delightful feelings.

57

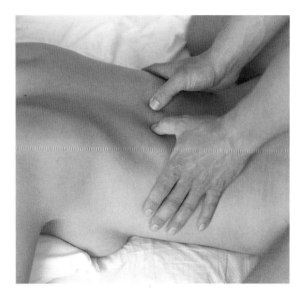

13. pressing the spine

From your position at the lower back, place your thumb pads on the bands of muscle running either side of the spine. Start to move your thumbs gently up the muscles, avoiding pressure, then press in where you feel tension or the muscles rise. You can use the thumbs very sensitively, keeping the pressure and withdrawal steady, taking care not to press directly on the spine. Releasing tension, this sparks sensations that travel through the whole body.

BACK INJURIES

While injuries should receive medical attention, you can ease problems as you massage. Do not massage directly over an injury, but work the surrounding area gently. Muscles around an injury often go into spasm to protect it. Massage can help relieve the stiffness caused by this, allowing the injury to heal. The body will often compensate to protect a painful area, so when the right shoulder hurts, you should also the work the left. shoulder. If the problem is caused by tension, work on and around the shoulder, easing the muscles outwards from the spine. Start lightly, then move in deeper, spreading and moving the shoulder frequently. For problems in the shoulders always include the lower back. For neck problems massage the upper back, then work on the neck from underneath. For the lower back, ease with sacral circling (see page 35), then massage the buttocks and middle back, spreading outwards from the spine.

14. completing the back

Having continued the pressure movements up either side of the spine, you need to change the pressure for the neck. As it will be turned, but is also extremely sensitive, a much softer movement is required. Use thumb and forefinger to press either side of the neck, reaching up to the very base of the skull. Releasing tension, this produces dreamy feelings. Leaving one hand at the neck, rest the other on the lower back to connect sensation down the spine (main picture).

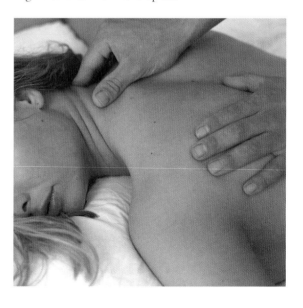

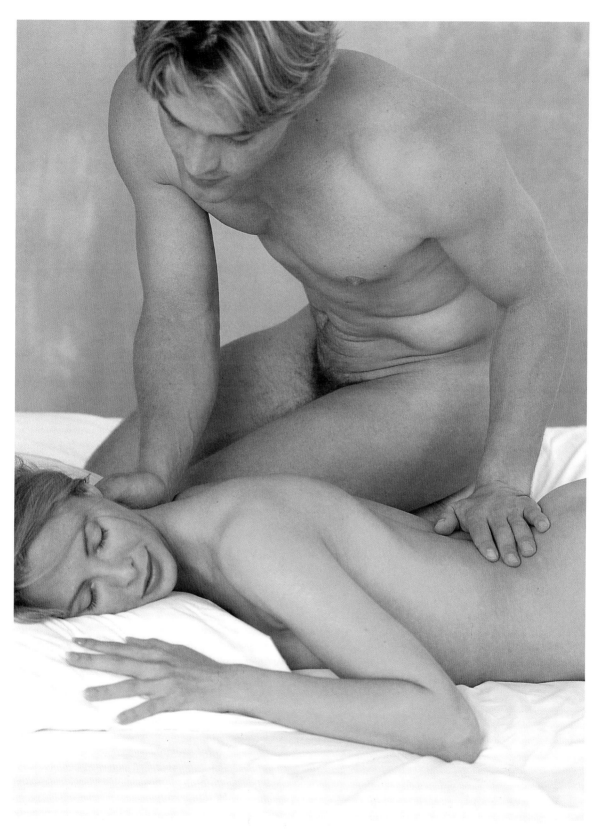

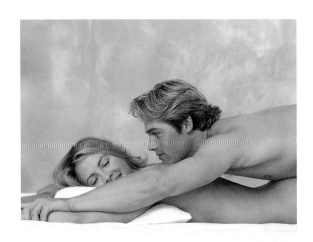

BACK TIPS

*A*fter following the structured massage sequence, why not spend some time being creative with your lover's back in other ways. It feels good to simply enjoy your partner's back, and feel her pleasure vibrating through the skin. Bring your body close to hers, and envelop her with a full body slide. The whole body contact feels great, and the fact that you can't get away from her back feels even better – for both of you! After the intensity of the massage, it feels good to relax, be playful, inventive and enjoy each other.

In a slightly more reflective mood, trace out every detail of your partner's back with small caresses. Her back, and the way you have come

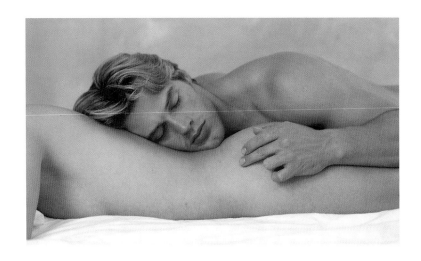

to know it, will surprise you. In massage, you come very close to your partner. Follow your instincts and if this is a good time to pause for a moment, be quiet together, and let your feelings merge. The softest moments and the smallest movements can often be the most intimate. Your lover's soft body curves provide a wonderful place to rest.

Blowing on the skin feels sensational. After the warm pressure of your hands during massage, the light, cool touch of your breath provides a beautiful contrast on the skin. Blow along the length of your partner's back and around the lower back curves. Bring your lips very close so the breath feels warmer, and watch the way the surface of the skin responds. Holding your partner continues the closeness of your contact, and enables you to brush her body with even more of your skin.

Try tracing gentle curves over your partner's skin with the backs of your hands. Idly stroke her over her body, in soft circles and curves, without stopping the rhythm of your hands. These gentle caresses feel very loving and warming.

Taking time to appreciate and admire your partner, seeing and feeling the difference as your massage progresses, the intimacy of the contact is such that there is almost no difference between you; your partner's body feels as familiar as your own. As for your partner, time loses all meaning in the bliss of endless variations of touch and delightful sensations.

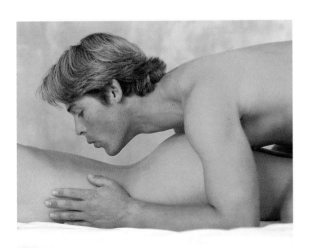
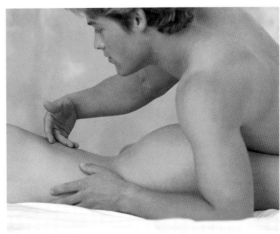

THE BACK OF THE LEGS

It is a natural progression of the sensual massage to now move your eyes down your partner's body to the legs. Notice their power, their length, the way they spread and the form of their muscles. Follow the contours around the thighs and buttocks, and the change in skin texture coming down to the feet. As the shape of the calves tapers towards the ankles, place your hands softly around the heels.

Of all the areas of the body, the legs often suffer the most neglect. For all the work they do in support and movement, our attention is so much more focused on the head and upper body, that, for some, awareness ends just below the hips. The legs and feet, however, are fully deserving of attention as they lead us forward toward new experiences.

GENERAL POINTS ABOUT LEG MASSAGE

When you effleurage the back of the legs you move from your partner's ankle up the calf to the thigh. Take care when you reach the back of the knee as it is very sensitive. So too is the inner thigh. Only gentle pressure should be used in these areas. You should brush only lightly if your partner has raised veins. Your partner will love the leg movements and stretches, but do not bend past the point of resistance. You should then ease the pressure once you reach this point. After massaging the legs, the movements for passive exercise (see pages 66-67) will help to stretch and tone the muscles and loosen the joints. Always aim for the optimum movement within your partner's range. Lowering your legs slowly and gently draws out exquisite feelings of release.

1. effleuraging the legs

Apply some more oil to your hands and kneel at your partner's feet. Then begin to effleurage one leg, starting at the ankle (main picture). Sweep up the leg to cover the back of the thigh and the buttock (left). You can effleurage the legs one at a time, or both at once, depending on your reach and balance. With the pressure on the upward stroke, keep the movement as one long sweep, allowing your hands to follow the curve and spread of your partner's muscles. Include the buttocks and hips as you stroke, as well as the sensitive, easily aroused inner thigh. Returning on the downward stroke, drag slightly with your fingertips around the back of the knee and calf, following the shape of the calf muscles. Tapering down with your fingers along the tendon to the heel, sweep around the feet and then return upwards to repeat the stroke. Apply a little bit more oil on your hands so that they glide easily over the legs.

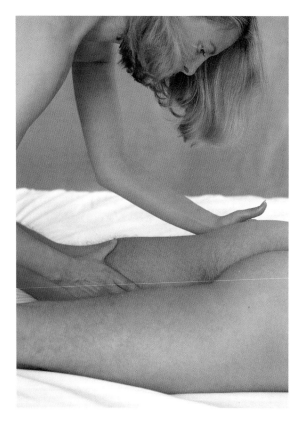

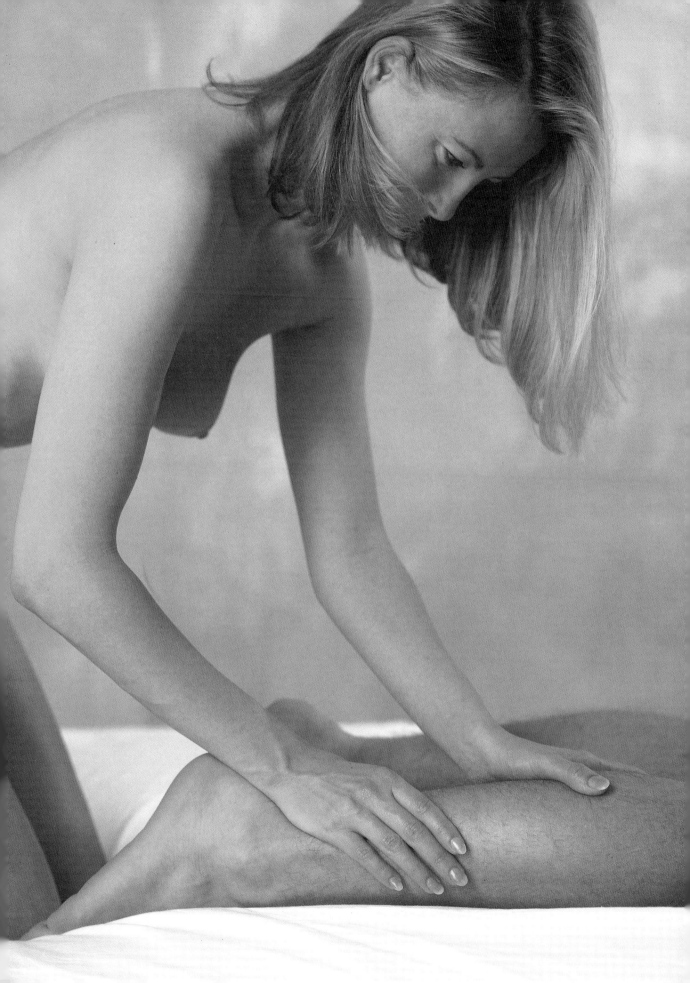

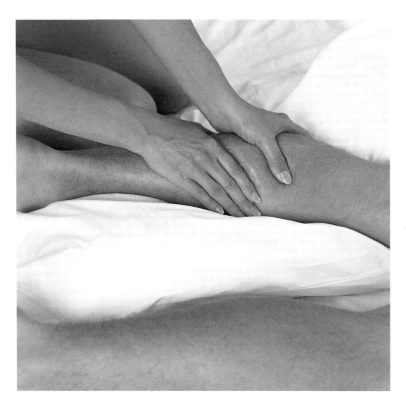

2. squeezing the calf

Returning to your partner's feet, form your hand into the tiger's mouth (see page 23), clasping the leg just above the ankle. With thumb and forefinger spread on either side, squeeze up the muscles as they swell to form the calf. Widen your hand as the muscles broaden, releasing the pressure as you near the knee. Squeezing movements like this help to remove toxins, in particular lactic acid. The build-up of toxins will be greater in well-formed muscles, so if this is the case, use both hands.

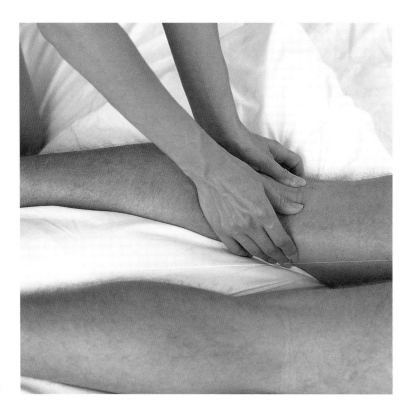

3. back of the knee

This is a wonderfully sensitive area that deserves special attention. Place the length of your thumbs in the center of the crease of your partner's knee. Keeping the pressure slight, slowly draw your thumbs apart. As your thumbs reach around the joint, lightly and slowly circle, dipping downwards, then sweeping up through the natural dimples. End the stroke with your thumbs trailing off up the back of the thigh.

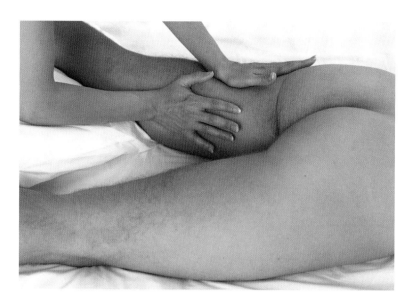

4. squeezing the thigh

To perform this, you may need to adjust your position, moving up to your partner's thigh. Use the flat of your hands to press firmly up the muscles, keeping the pressure light on the sensitive inner thigh. If the leg muscles are particularly strong, use the heels of your hands to press up the back and the outer thigh. Continue pressure towards the buttock, moving across and over the hip.

ABOUT THE LEGS

The legs not only contain the longest bone in the body, the femur, but also one of its most complicated joints, the knee. The sciatic nerve, the body's largest peripheral nerve, passes down through the pelvis and back of the leg to the foot. Usually, any pain in this nerve has a connection in the lower back. The leg muscles are particularly powerful, with three long muscles (the hamstrings) running down the backs of the thighs. The feet provide both mobility and stable support, but it is the bones of the leg that directly bear the body's weight. The legs are extremely powerful and highly sensitive. The backs and sides of the thigh are responsive to firm pressure, while the inner thigh and buttock are more delicate. The feelings aroused here can be very erotic. The calf muscles enjoy reasonably firm touch, but for a woman, it may need to be quite light. Check with your partner. The feet and ankles delight in massage and movement, enjoying the unaccustomed freedom it brings.

5. stroking the thigh

With the backs of your fingers, stroke up, along the thighs toward the buttocks. As the backs of the fingers are very sensitive, this movement will also be enjoyable for you. Keep the pressure light enough to sensitize and arouse, but for a man especially, not soft enough to tickle. End the strokes curling over the buttocks, sending sensations right up the spine.

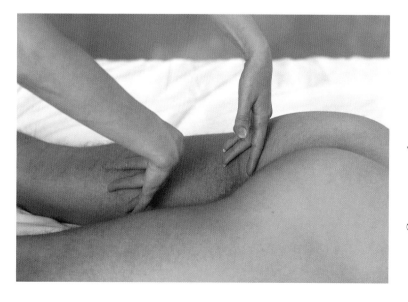

A FULL SENSUAL MASSAGE – *the back of the legs*

65

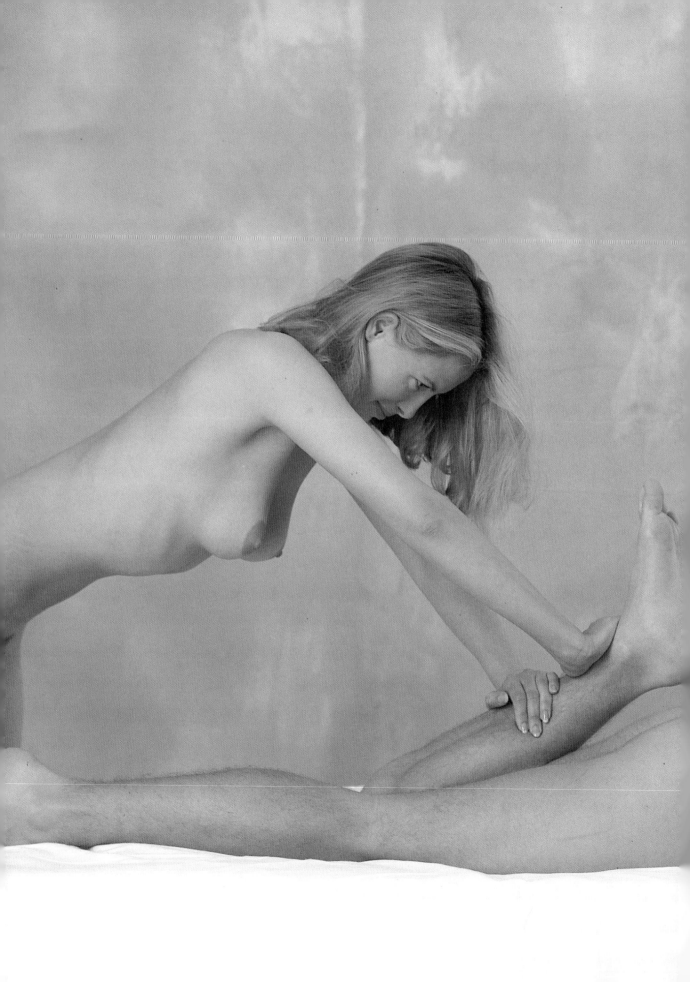

6. stretch and circle

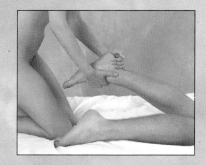

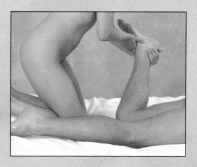

With broad, deep, enthusiastic strokes, begin kneading the back of your partner's thigh (below). Keep the pressure at the back and side, working only lightly over the inner area where the leg artery runs. Twist and roll the flesh to loosen up the muscles, freeing the thigh for sensations that run right down to the feet. Stroking gently back down the leg, place one hand over

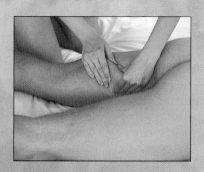

the heel and one around the front of the foot. Then lifting the leg slightly, pull back toward you, giving a stretch that can be felt in the lower back and hips (above). Raise the leg and begin to circle it slowly, several times in one direction, then several times in the other direction (above right). Take the whole leg weight, holding the foot and ankle for support, and only circle it well within your

partner's range. Felt in the hip and knee joints, this movement gives a satifying roll to the muscles at the back of the thigh. For a final releasing stretch along the front of the thigh, press the leg back, heel toward the buttock (main picture). Applying pressure gradually through the arms, press until you feel the leg resist. Then lower it gently, keeping contact with your hands.

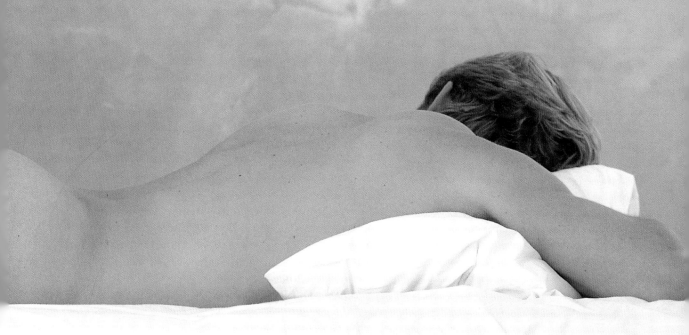

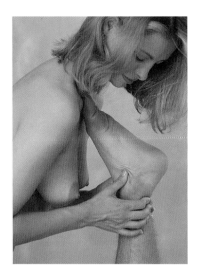
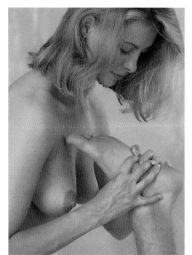

7. *completing the legs*

Bringing your partner's leg back toward you, begin to work deeply around the ankle joint (far left). Using your thumbs, circle slowly and evenly on both sides, working close to the bone. Now, move down to the foot. Support it from underneath with your thumbs. Interlace your fingers across the sole, then slowly start to draw them apart (left). This action spreads the foot, leading to a sense of freedom and expansion. Ease the pressure as you reach the sides of the foot, cupping your hands around the instep and ankle joint. Do this movement several times over. Lowering the leg to rest on your thigh as a support, press over the sole of the foot with your thumbs (bottom left). Using a reasonably firm pressure, press with the pads to cover the entire foot. This creates a wonderfully releasing movement, which reaches down the entire body. Keep the pressure and withdrawal slow and steady, to increase the hypnotic rhythm and sheer delight. Then place the foot down gently, and start the entire sequence on the other leg. While your partner's body pulses with exquisite sensations, close the back of the leg massage by resting for a moment or so, while you hold your partner's feet (main picture). This time of stillness is beneficial to both of you.

HEAD TO TOE AWARENESS

Completing the massage at the feet gives immediate satisfaction. As reflex zones of the feet relate to all the organs of the body, massage here can revitalize the whole system and seems to penetrate the very bones. At the end of the massage, pause to rest and to allow the sensations flooding over your partner's body to diffuse.

Massaging the back of the body provides strength and support for the vulnerable front. With the entire back of the body relaxed and alive with sensation, finish off with gentle brushstrokes to bring awareness from head to toe.

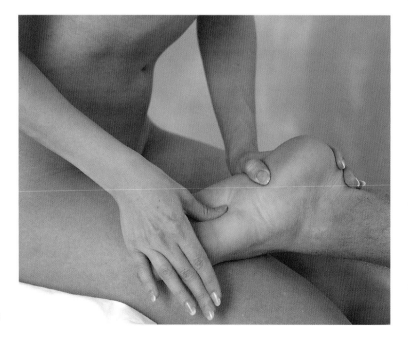

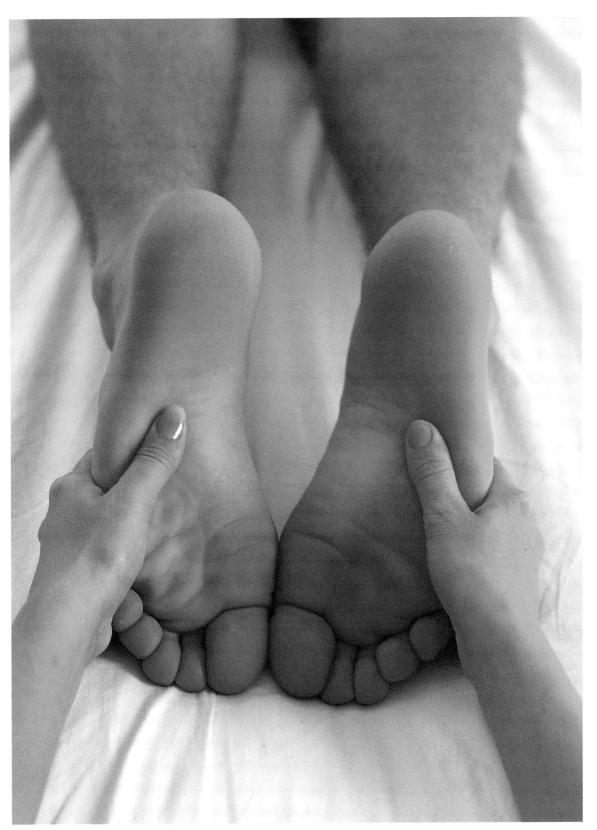

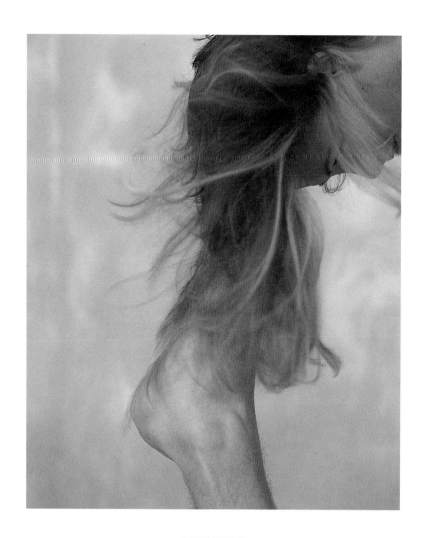

LEG TIPS

*T*he legs feel and look wonderful when they are relaxed and supple. After the leg massage, take some time to explore a variety of sensations and sensual movements with your partner.

The soles of the feet are very sensitive, and can often be ticklish, but they are extremely responsive to touch. Play with your partner's toes: they can be very erogenous. They can also be a source of great pleasure and childish laughter. For an interesting sensual feel, try stimulating your partner's feet with your hair. Brush softly with your hair all over the foot, or, if your partner can take it and your hair is long enough, flick the ends at the soles of his feet. Short, sharp flicks can be very arousing. It also feels good to your partner to lose his foot amongst your hair!

Leg movement can be very graceful. Leg to leg, sole to sole, brings the legs together, concentrating feeling and contact through the feet. Use the sensitivity of your feet to feel each other, experimenting with the different shapes your legs create. For playful movement, you can bicycle the legs together, pushing and stretching to feel the angle of your limbs. Feel the sensations you produce as you press and move against one another, using the soft, sensitive pads of your feet.

Take time getting to know your partner's legs intimately. Brush against them with your entire body, or softly caress them with your toes. Slowly feel their entire length with your feet. Gently blowing between the toes feels very sensual, separating each one and giving a little pull. Rub your legs, hip to hip or back to back, feeling every detail of your partner's skin.

The natural result of massaging the body is that it becomes more integrated, a complete whole once again. Movements are spontaneous and expressive; it is almost as if you have become re-acquainted with your limbs. Moving the legs, when they feel connected to the back, is completely relaxed and effortless. Express the pleasure in your legs together with your partner, sharing the enjoyment of how good they feel. Get to know your partner's body through your legs, keeping the contact intimate and special.

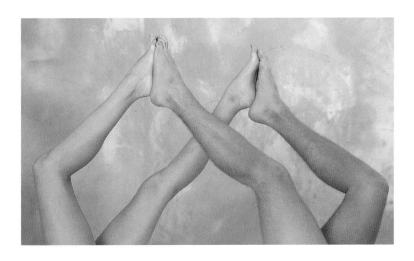

THE NECK

With your partner lying on her back, you should position yourself at her head, with your knees on either side. Before beginning work on the neck, take a moment to be sensitive to your partner's body. The front of the body is naturally more vulnerable and open than the back, and your massage should reflect this. See the soft, relaxed roundness in the way the body lies, from the swell of the breasts to the abdomen, hips and legs. Note the delicate facial features, the muscles of the neck and then concentrate your full attention on the shoulders and gently bring your hands toward your partner's chest.

The neck often carries a lot of tension, so in this position the muscles are resting naturally, without having to support the head. A soft, releasing massage on the neck muscles immediately affects the upper back. The most important muscles for neck massage are the 'trapezius' (at the back of the neck), and the 'sternolcleidomastoid' (at the side), which turns the head. The cervical vertebrae supporting the head form a natural spinal curve. If the neck is lengthened through stretching, a feeling of release reverberates down the spine.

The sweeping effleurage strokes you use around the breasts and ribs will connect

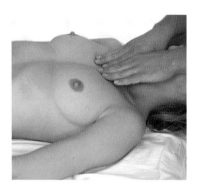 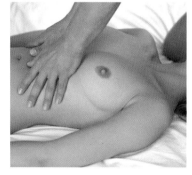 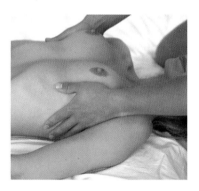

1. effleurage and stretch
Rub more oil onto your fingers. Begin the massage by placing your fingertips lightly on your partner's chest (above), then sweep down with your hands between her breasts. Spread your hands to follow the curve of your partner's body, sweeping your fingers round the ribs (above center). As you turn your hands, press the flesh firmly, then slowly pull up the side of the body (above right). Drag

slightly with your fingertips. Curve your hands to dip around the shoulders, then sliding round behind the shoulders, stretch down and away from you with the heels (below right). Continue by sweeping up the back of the neck, until your fingers are under the base of the skull. Complete the movement by stretching up and back towards you, lengthening the neck and releasing tension in the spine (main picture). Pull off

through the hair and gently lower the head. Complete this movement several times, using luxurious, gliding strokes.

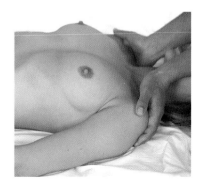

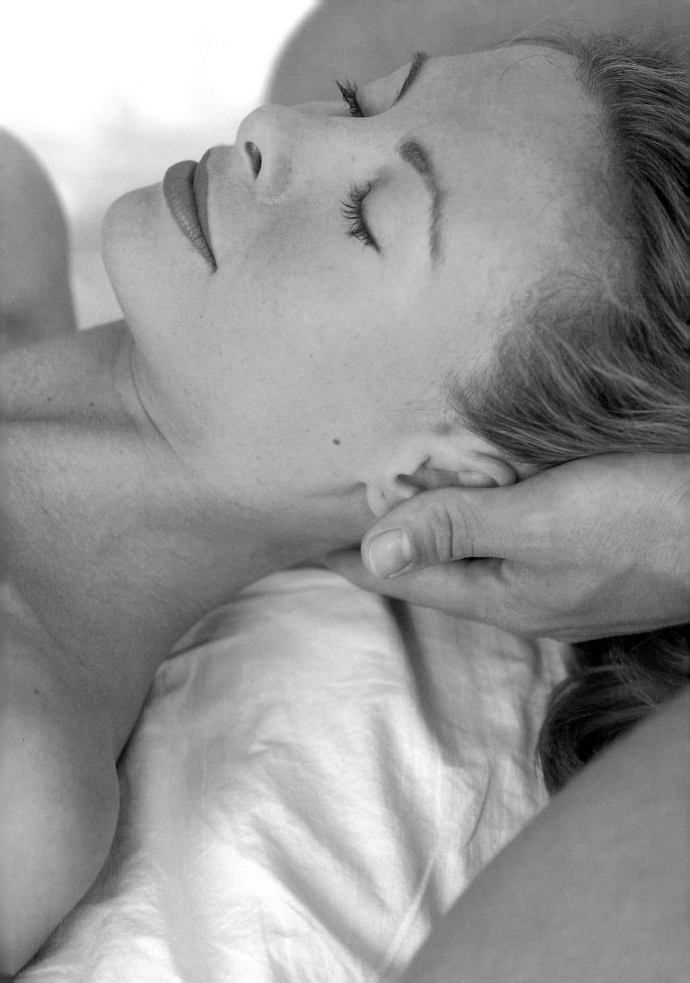

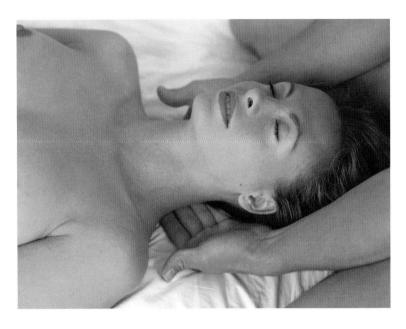

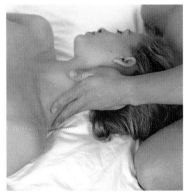

2. rolling

Roll the head from side to side. Then with your hands beneath the neck, make small circles up the muscles on either side. Use your fingertips to work lightly from the base toward the skull (above left). Turn the head, and after pushing the shoulder down, smooth up the neck with the flat of your hand (above). As you reach the base of the skull, press in and under with your fingertips, keeping the pressure slow and even (below left). Tousle and shampoo your partner's hair (below), then finger up to the ends (main picture).

sensations from the torso to the neck. In fact as you stretch the neck and push the shoulders, the whole upper torso begins to release. Including the movements of the relaxation massage (see pages 38-39), bring your hands to the back of the neck, and use small circles to release. Pressing slowly at the base of the neck releases tension, at the same time increasing sensuality. To end the massage, relax the scalp and tousle your partner's hair, tugging gently at the roots with your fingertips.

It is only after releasing the neck that we feel a wonderful sense of freedom, the body almost flooding with euphoria. It is no exaggeration to say that a soft, relaxed neck creates a softer and more open state of mind.

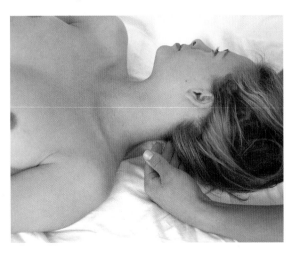

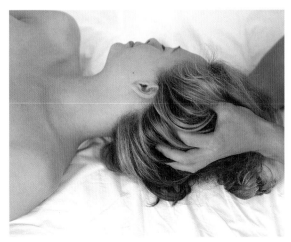

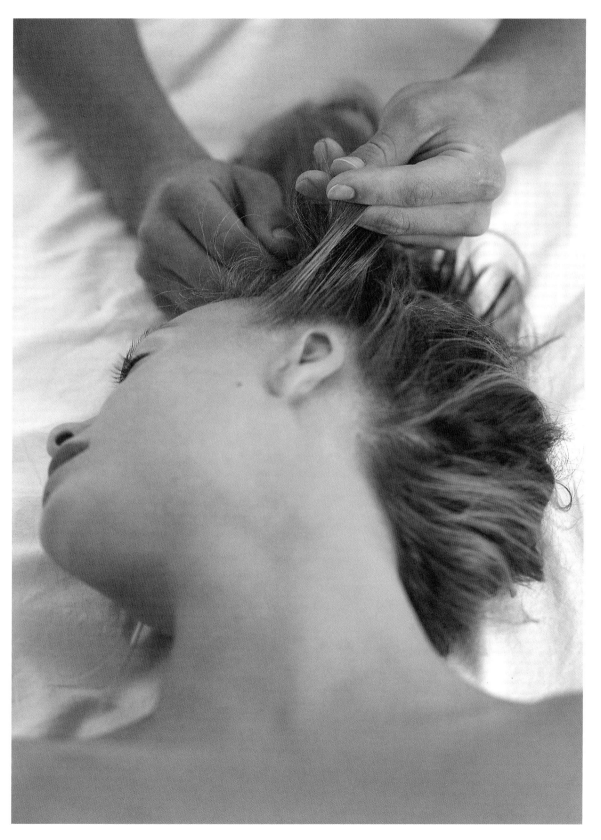

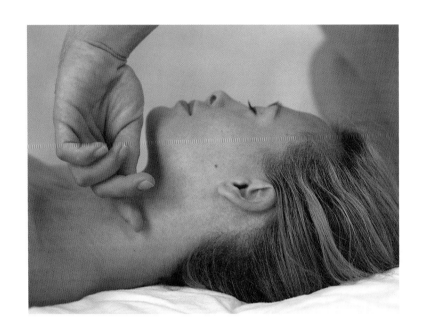

NECK TIPS

*T*he neck and throat areas are extremely delicate and sensitive. This makes them extremely responsive to sensation. Using a tender, delicate touch will fully open up your partner's senses.

With the sensitive backs of your fingertips, trace lightly up your partner's throat. Follow every detail, softly drawing up and under the chin. As your touch continues almost imperceptibly, the entire body will be

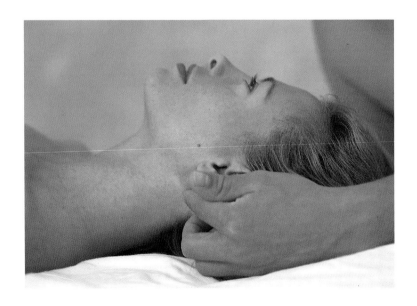

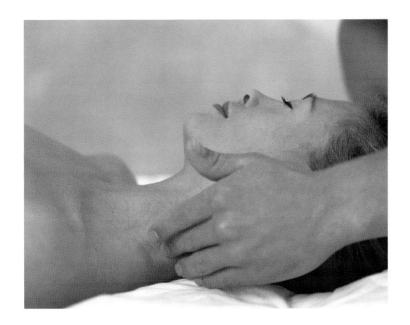

awash with sensation. Or you can gently brush with your forefinger around the crescent of the ear following the curve back and forth. The skin behind the ear is very soft and delicate. Stimulate it with the pads of your fingers, playing softly along the line of the hair. More wonderful sensations are produced by you brushing up the side of her neck with your fingers. Start stroking in the sensitive hollow above the collar bone, and pull softly upwards until you reach the dimple behind the ear. This sends tingles over the skin, down the spine and around the scalp. Watch to see the goose bumps on your partner's flesh. Choose a few strands of hair from the highly sensitive nape of your partner's neck, then gently tease and pull the hairs, keeping them taut between your fingers. Draw out the sensation by pulling the very ends.

Exploring your partner's body, watching closely the way she responds, increases the feeling between you of tenderness and intimacy. It is a whole new pleasure to find ways to please your partner, providing different sensations for her to experience. As you touch your partner's body, share your experiences, how her body feels to you and how your touch feels to her.

THE FACE

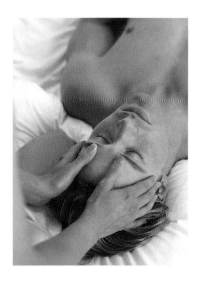

After the neck and scalp have been massaged and are tingling, turn your attention to the face. By gently massaging the face, you can send glowing feelings all through your partner's head. Beginning at the forehead, rest your hands for a moment, and tune into your partner's state of mind.

The delicate muscles of the face are constantly used to reflect the way we feel, but they can become quite tight. Tension over the forehead, around the eyes, and especially round the jaw prohibits fluidity of facial expression. The mouth, a highly mobile structure, is very sensual, and the nerve endings are extremely sensitive to touch. The forehead, when we feel calm, is relaxed and smooth. Our eyes tell the world how we feel.

1. releasing strokes

Smooth a little oil over your fingers. Then place the length of your thumbs in the center of your partner's forehead, your hands cupped gently around the head (above). Draw your thumbs apart, gradually and evenly, releasing the pressure as you curve round

to the temples. Dipping your thumbs to circle round the temples, bring the movement back, and draw out across the eyebrows (below left). Without breaking the continuity, place the pads of your thumbs just below the eye-socket ridge. Start from the outer edge, then press gently along the muscles,

using tiny movements at even intervals round to the nose (below right). Moving your thumbs to rest across the cheekbones, smooth your hands over the cheeks and pull up toward the ears (main picture). Cup your hands gently around the face and spread the muscles upwards into a smile.

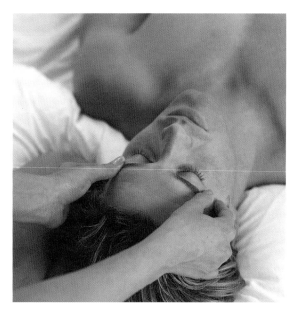

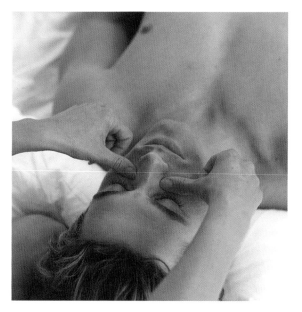

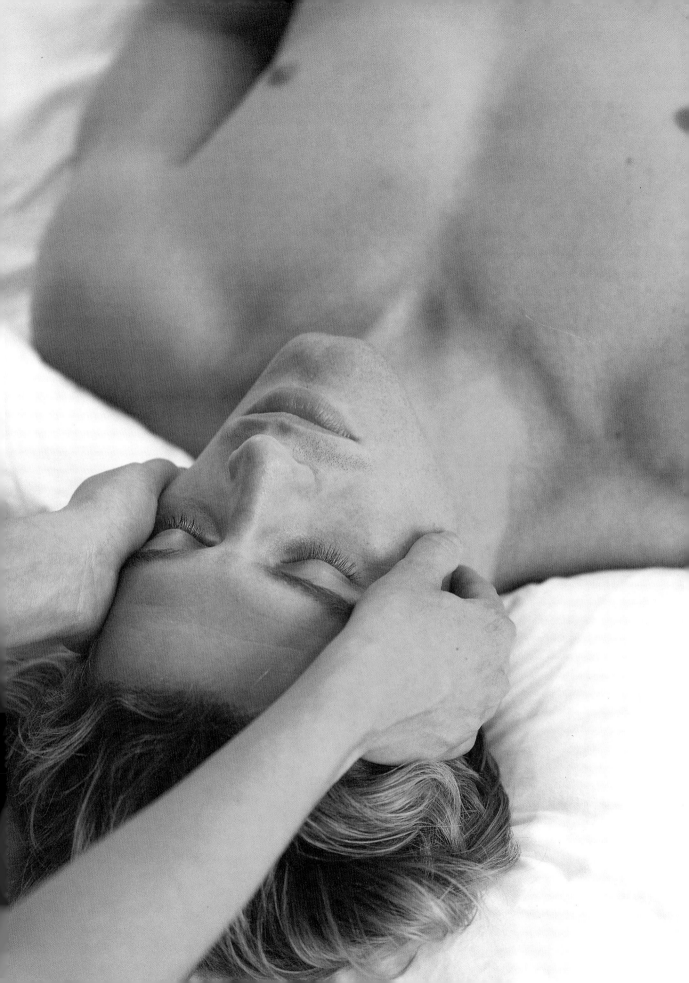

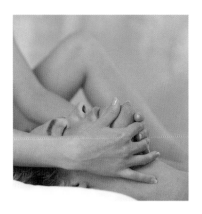 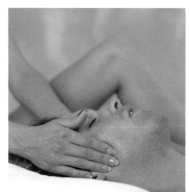

It is only when someone actually massages the face that we become aware of how much the muscles are used. As you smooth across your partner's forehead, any tightness will start to diffuse, the feeling spreading as you work around the eyes. Smoothing over the cheeks and around the chin restores feeling and flexibility, completed by broad circling movements to release the jaw. The jaw, which can become clenched tightly, should hang just slightly open, with the tongue relaxed at the bottom of the mouth. By now your partner's face will feel blissfully released – the experience reaches too deep to even talk. Often, it can feel as if a mask has been taken off to reveal a pure state of natural expression.

Complete the massage with loving touches to your partner's features, stroking down the nose and tracing lightly with your fingertips around the mouth. Gentle squeezing and pulling of the earlobes can feel quite wonderful.

2. circling and brushing

Interlace your fingers under the chin, then pull them apart, spreading up the line of the jaw (above left). Keeping your thumbs above and your forefingers below the jaw line, slide round and upwards until you reach the joint. To release any tightness in the area, ask your partner to slightly drop his jaw, then make slow, broad circles with your fingertips (above right). Softly brush your thumb along the length of your partner's nose, using rolling strokes from the bridge to the very tip (below left). Repeat this several times, following the curve to reach his lips (below right). Trace lightly with your fingertips around the mouth. To continue stimulation of your partner's senses, squeeze and tug the earlobes between your finger and thumb (main picture). Slide down to the lobes, brushing with your lips.

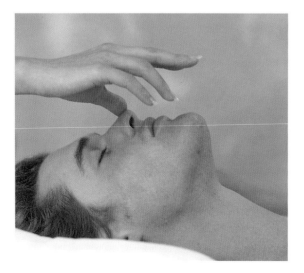 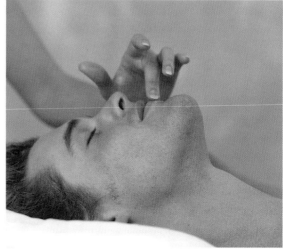

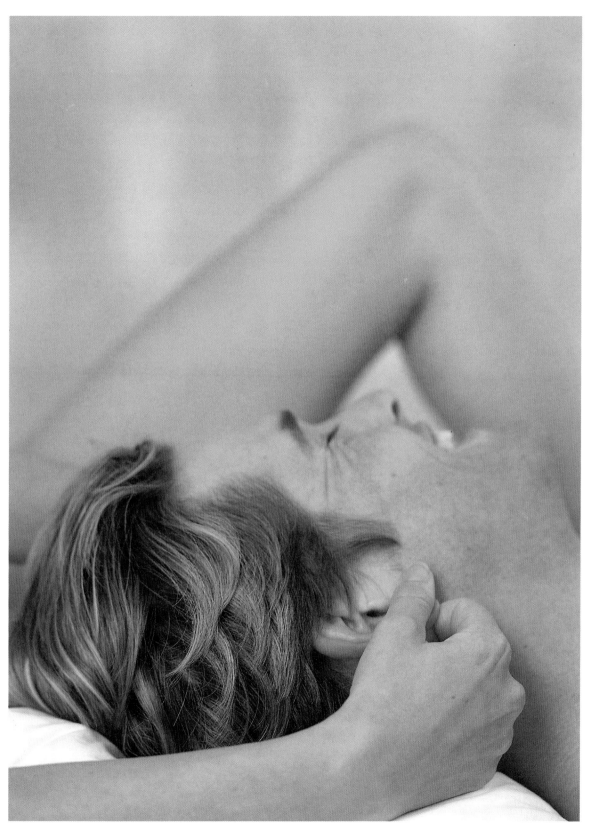

THE ARMS

By now relaxation and sensual pleasure will be seeping down your partner's body. You need to move to his side to begin massage on the arms. Look for a moment to absorb each area in detail, following from the shoulder to the slimness of the wrists. Note the way your partner rests his forearm, then bring your eyes to the powerful, sensitive hands. Make soft initial contact at the wrist, then begin the sweep of effleurage strokes up the arms.

When you massage the arms, bear in mind that, like the legs, you can do each part of the massage alternating between the two arms or you can massage one at a time. When you begin work on the inner arm, be aware of the exquisitely sensitive skin on the inner elbow. Take a few moments to sense out the area with your fingertips, stimulating and arousing as you stroke. The movements on the arm should flow into one another, progressing rhythmically up towards the shoulder. Firm pressure along the upper arm releases the bulk of the muscles, which often become tight and solid. Use the flat of your hand to press and smooth around the armpit, keeping the pressure sensitive yet firm as you explore the dips

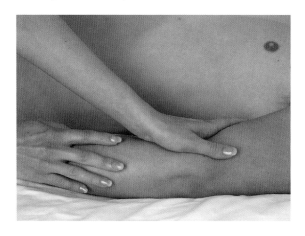 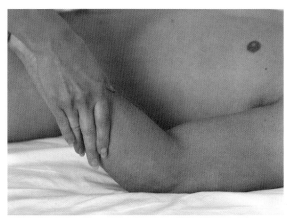

1. effleurage and squeezing

Apply some oil to your hands, then use effleurage strokes in full gliding movements up the arm (above left). Be sure to oil right up over the shoulder. Gently rock the arm between your hands as you return to loosen any tension. You should only use pressure on the upward stroke. Keep the strokes flowing, free and generous sliding and turning on the lighter

downward stroke. Do this movement several times, then lifting the arm at the wrist (above right), squeeze up the forearm muscles with the tiger's mouth (see page 23). Use the forefinger joint and thumb for extra pressure. Work the length of the muscles right up to the elbow, squeezing as you release the pressure to work round the elbow joint (main picture). As you press, you will be

giving your partner a feeling of deep release, sending wonderful tingling sensations down the whole length of the arms. Press sensitively with your thumb, and feel around the bones, trailing off with small circling movements at the back of the upper arm. As you perform this movement, be careful of the 'ulnar' nerve, situated at the back of the elbow and often known as the funny bone.

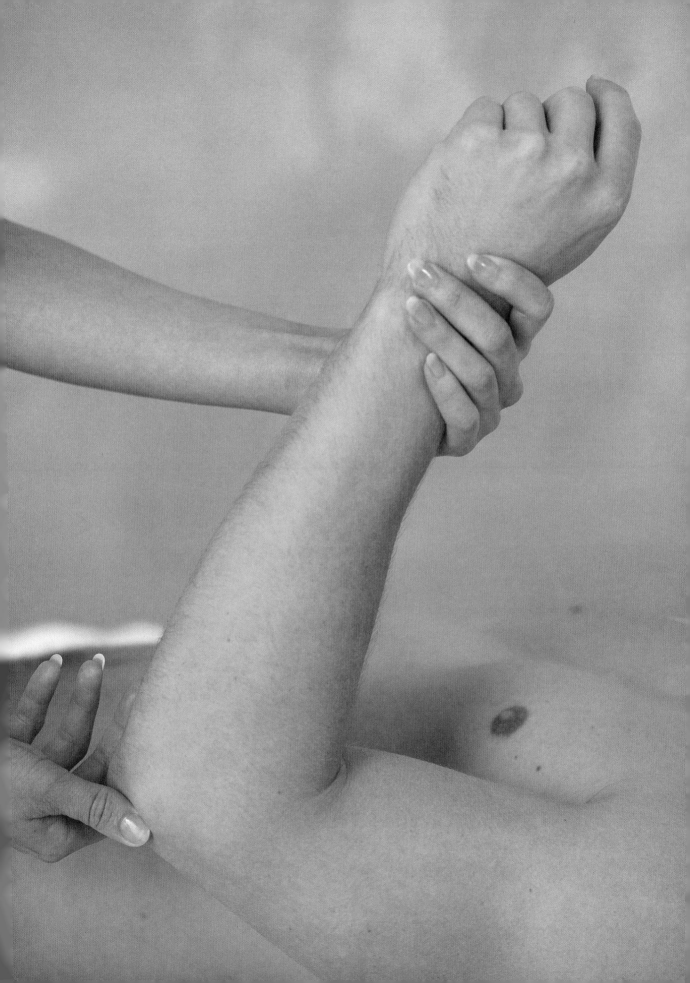

2. the inner arm and elbow

Lower your partner's forearm once again, then turn the palm over, supporting the forearm at the wrist. With the flat of your hand, begin smoothing up the inner arm muscles, pressing with reasonable firmness towards the elbow (below left). Sweep round the arm to the wrist, as you return and without breaking the rhythm of your hands, slide up the arm again, exerting some pressure. This will feel both soothing and sensual to your partner and produces a delightful tingling in his palm. Repeat these strokes several times. Afterwards, turn your attention to the inner elbow, and use your fingertips to brush along the crease (below right). This is a very sensitive area and feels wonderful as you stroke along the line of the elbow joint. Use your fingers to stimulate, or, dragging along the crease, dip and circle them along the outer edge. Spend several moments here. As you linger over the skin, this will totally mesmerize your partner.

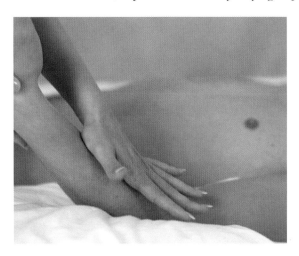 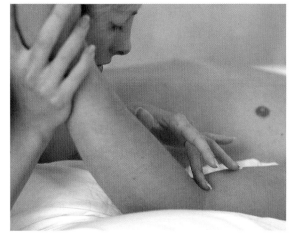

and curves. Circling movements, followed by slowly releasing the pressure, can have a delightfully erotic feel. A full stretch of your partner's arm is wonderfully releasing, both freeing the arm and having an effect right down the spine (see page 86). The feeling of someone else stretching your limbs is an unusual, extremely pleasurable experience. As you press down the forearm, moving to the wrist, be aware of the delicate structure. As you circle very gently with your fingertips you can feel the minute detail of the bones. The hands deserve a good deal of attention, being used, almost unconsciously, every second of the day. Without realizing it a lot of tension can build here, only coming to a person's attention when they are receiving a massage on the hands. Spend time caressing and releasing every inch of your partner's fingers, then, after brushstrokes, tenderly entwine them in your own. Just allow the fingers to idly touch and play as a sweet, loving gesture of affection.

ABOUT THE ARMS

Our arms play an important part in our self-expression, as well as being indispensable for work. It is with our arms that we draw people and objects closer, and equally use them to push those things away. We naturally use our arms for our protection, while our hands demonstrate what we say and express the way we feel. We use our hands to manipulate

3. the upper arm

Now lift your partner's arm to place it at a right angle across the body, and give the forearm support by holding it at the wrist (below left). Then cup your other hand around the upper arm muscles, and press firmly down toward the shoulder. Squeeze the muscles tightly, following their roundness,

using pressure between your heel and fingers. Apply the movement to both outer and inner arm muscles, using your thumbs for extra strength. As you reach the shoulder, slide your hand around the joint. Then supporting the upper arm with both hands, lower it behind your partner's head. Using the flat of your hand, press

lightly round the armpit (below right). Pressing sensitively around the curves and hollows, this movement feels deliciously sensual. If your partner is ticklish, start lightly but firmly, and then increase the pressure. Press and circle using different points of your hands, ending by soft brushstrokes up the arm toward the elbow.

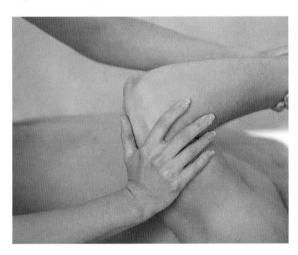
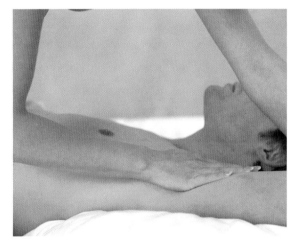

objects, make things or be creative. We hold out our hands to invite contact with another person, and of course, we use our hands for touch. The fingertips are extremely sensitive, and pick up numerous messages that tell us about the world. The palms of the hands, also very sensitive, are an area from where we issue strength.

The bones of the forearm are so arranged that in order for the arm to turn, one bone rotates around the other. Pressure between the bones can feel extremely good. The wrist provides a fulcrum for movement of the hands, which is facilitated by the structure of the finger joints. Passive movement of these joints always feels beneficial. The nerves supplying

the arms originate from the neck, so massage around the neck and shoulders often travels down the length of the arms. The biceps and triceps are the strong upper arm muscles, effecting the movements of the forearm. Interacting with the upper arm, muscles in the back and upper chest facilitate movement of the mobile shoulder joint.

Arm movements are an extension of the body, and, flowing and expansive, come from around the shoulder blades. If the chest is also relaxed and open, this releases energy down the arms. The arm position and movements are affected if the chest feels tight, contracted and held in. When the arms are free, they suddenly feel more sensitive and much lighter.

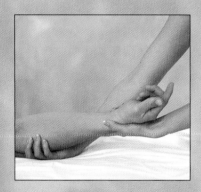

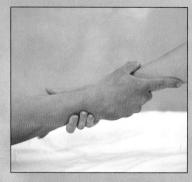

3. stretch and circle

Positioning yourself behind your partner's head, bend forwards to take hold of his arm. With one hand around the hand and the other supporting the elbow, gently pull the length of the arm back toward you (main picture). Start the stretch slowly, increasing the pull until you feel resistance, then ease the pressure. Your partner will feel the stretch around the ribs and upper back. As you perform the stretch, take care not to compromise your spine, leaning back with the weight of your body. You can experiment with the position of your hold, supporting the forearm or wrist or gripping your partner's arm (above left and right). To make the stretch more active for your partner, he can also entwine his grip around your own. So your partner feels a satisfying stretch, make sure he is relaxed and gives you his full arm weight. As you put your whole body behind your action, this movement will feel equally good for you. To lower the arm, keep supporting with your hands and circle it round to the side (below). Then with his upper arm resting, but still holding the forearm, gently lower the arm to your partner's side.

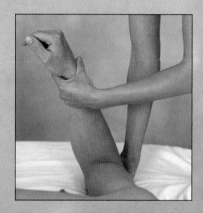

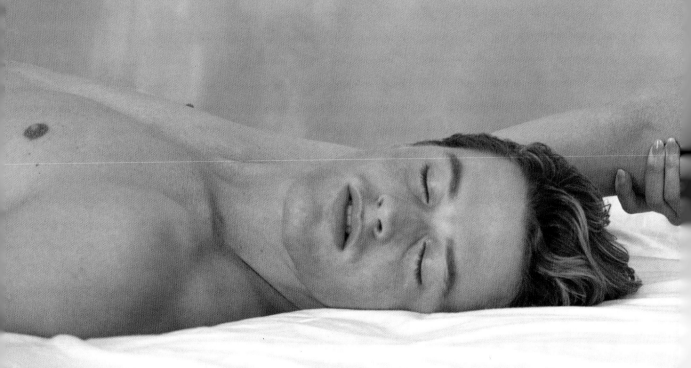

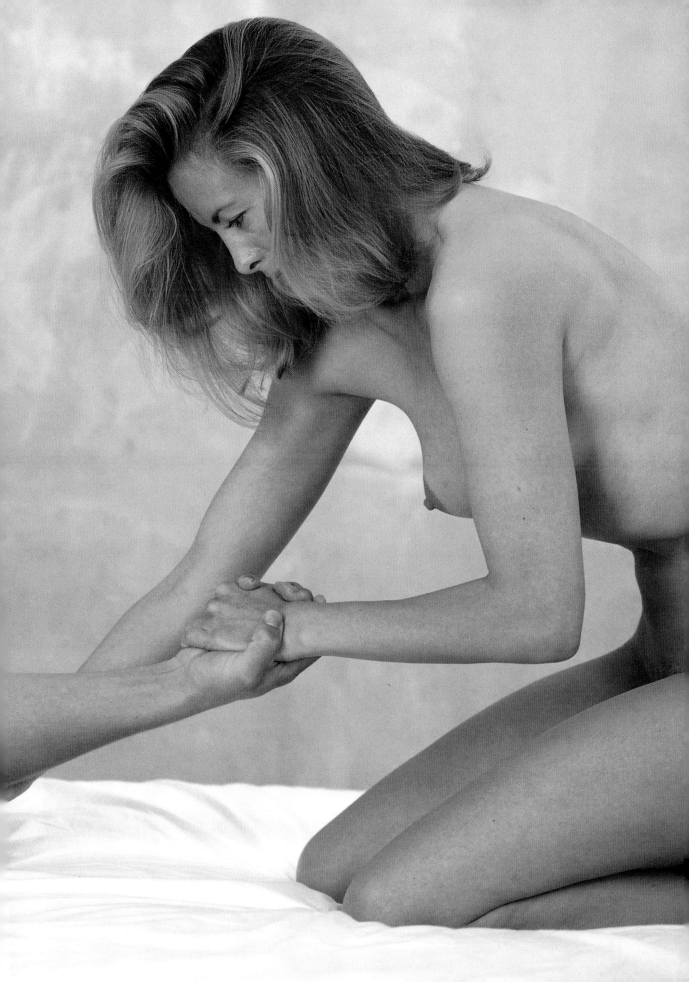

PREVENTING TENSION IN THE ARMS

As you are massaging your partner's arms, note any differences you feel between the left and the right. For people who are right handed, for example, the right side will tend to be more developed and probably more tense. The right side of the body is primarily controlled by the rational and logical left side of the brain, while the creative, intuitive right side of the brain influences the left side of the body. Very often tension in the arms and shoulders relates to the ways we use our minds. It is important to keep an even balance between activities, and to use both sides of the body. For example, if you are right-handed, keep your left side active. Try and do things with both hands. As a general rule, after muscles have been working, give them time to relax.

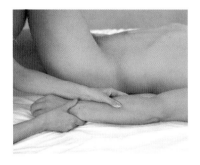
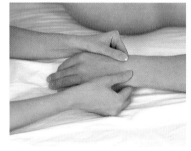
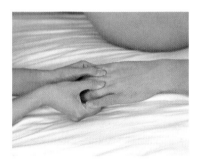

4. completing the arms

Holding the wrist, press evenly but firmly with the length of your thumb down the center of your partner's forearm (above left). As you reach the wrist, use both thumbs to press and make small circles around the bones of the joint (above center). Moving outwards

from the center, work your way across the wrist, sliding round to draw down between the tendons of the hand (above right). Pull slowly, drawing tension out between the fingers, then turn the hand and circle over the palm with your thumbs (below left). The pressure can be quite firm to feel

fully satisfying, while a light stretch between the fingers enhances the sensation. Press, twist and squeeze as you pull tantalizingly off each finger (below right). Then repeat the sequence on the other arm. End gently with soft caresses with your fingers (main picture).

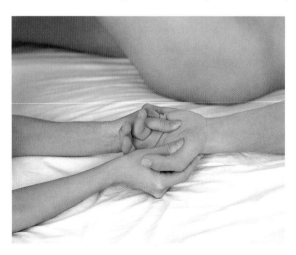
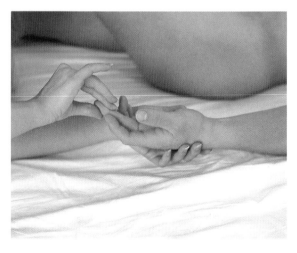

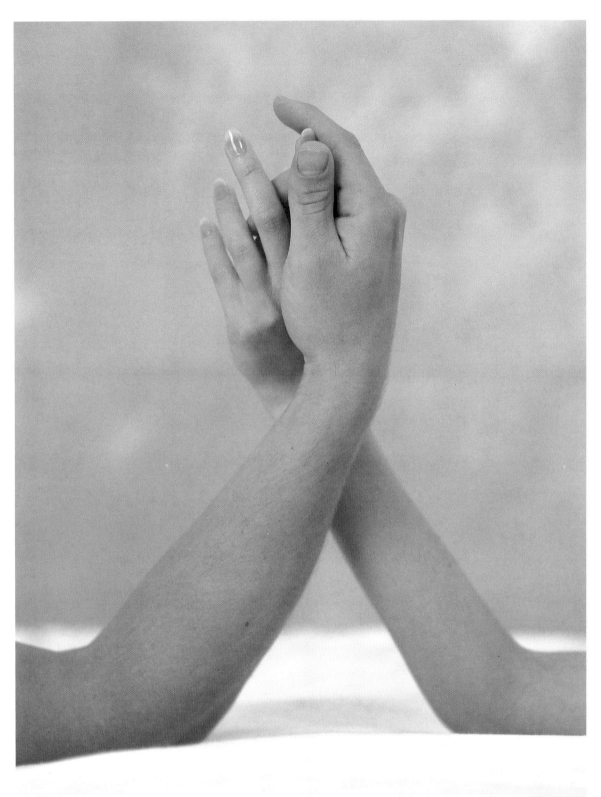

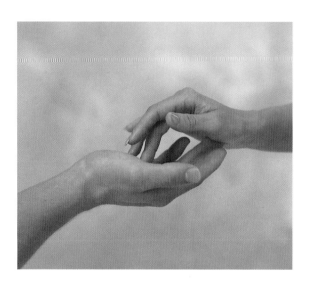

ARM TIPS

*A*s your partner basks in the warmth of the feelings running through his arms, now released, relaxed and sensitized, it is the perfect time for more sensual discovery.

With your partner's hand turned up toward you, make the gentlest of movements across the palm. Touching and stroking lightly with your fingertips, circle and explore the hand. Trace with your fingers along the lines, closely feeling every fold and crease. Like the face, the hands reflect our world experience, and the way they have been used through a person's life. Close your eyes and let your fingers discover for you. You will feel your partner in a completely different way.

Using your nails can be an erotically arousing experience. With the tip of your nail, draw across your partner's wrist. The heel of the hand and inner wrist are very sensitive, so there need only be a hint of pressure. Follow up the inside of your partner's arm, drawing with the nail to the sensitive elbow crease. Keeping the touch intriguingly light and delicate, nails add a dimension to sensation for your partner.

Explore different ways you can touch each other's arms and hands, using the tip of the nails and fingers, or drawing along the edge. Explore the shape and movement of the forearm, the sensation of the pulse at the wrist. Move up the arm, and feel the contours as the arm rounds into the shoulder. Circle around the uneven and neglected elbow, and return to the familiar roundness of the fingertips. Use your fingers as an extension of your eyes.

For a change in sensation, blow softly on the palm, altering the shape of your mouth to change the impact of the breath. Or circle with your elbow in the center of the palm, which has a surprising effect of spreading warmth. Caress your partner's arms using your outer forearm, then feel out your partner's body with the backs of your wrists and hands.

As you embrace, be aware of the soft quality in the ways you use your arms. The arms can be used to hold each other close, to encircle and cherish the things we value. If you are still and simply hold your partner's hand be aware of the feelings that go back and forwards between you.

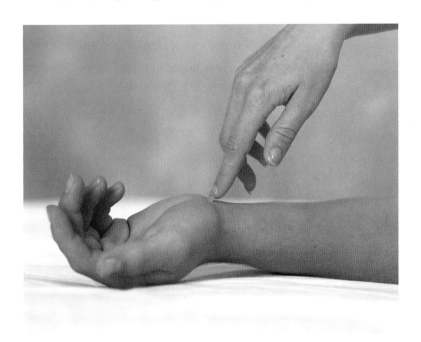

THE CHEST

Sit at your partner's head to finish the massage on the upper body. Before starting the massage look at your partner's body, look at the sensitivity of the breasts, at the openness of the chest, the ribs, the abdomen.

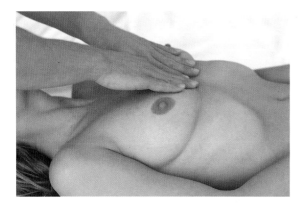

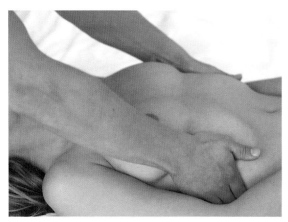

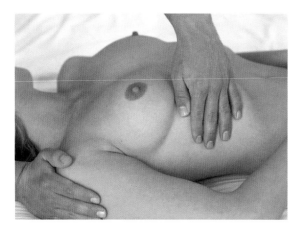

During the massage you will be using both the effleurage technique and stretch to open up the body, pulling up around the ribs and breasts to expand and release the chest.

The main muscles for massage are the pectorals, whose movements are connected to the back. The ribcage, protecting the vital heart and lungs, is also important to massage. The intercostal muscles (between the ribs) work together with the diaphragm, so that the ribcage expands as we breathe in. When breathing is relaxed, the upper chest remains almost still. The breath reaches right to the abdomen when the body breathes naturally.

Feel your partner's vulnerability and sensitivity by placing your hand over the center of her chest. As the heart pumps blood around the body, massage assists the flow of blood. Keep the strokes sensitive, caressing your partner's body with loving, sensual touches.

1. effleurage and release

Re-oiling your hands, begin the massage with full effleurage strokes over your partner's chest. Slip down over the breastbone, avoiding pressure to the breasts (above left) and glide your hands over and around the ribs, pulling up just under your partner's body (center left). Give a deep stretch along the ribs, curving your hands softly around the breasts. Return to the top of the chest and complete the movement several times. Then, resting one hand on your partner's shoulder, place the other just under the ribs. Pull up and across toward you (below left), sweeping your hand around the shape of the breast. Then push over the pectoral muscles (situated just above the breast), ending the movement at the arm (main picture). Repeat the movement on the other side.

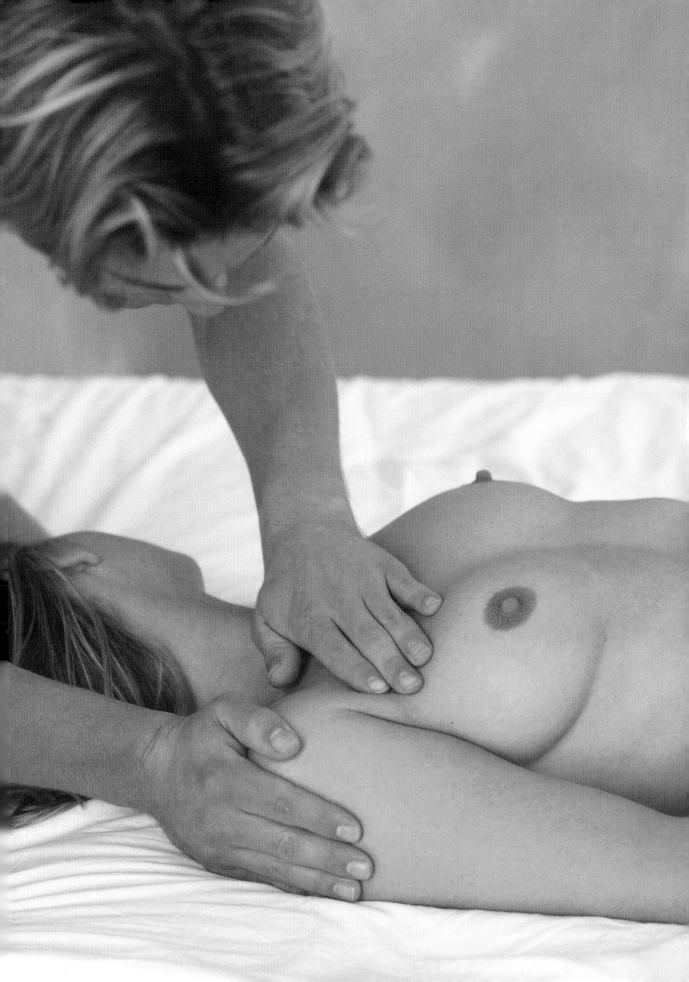

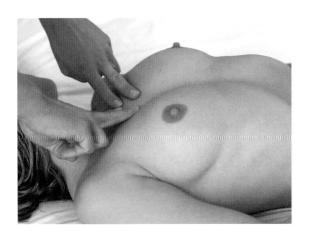

2. release along the ribs

Place your first two fingers in the center of the chest, on either side of the breastbone. With your forefingers under the first rib, and your second fingers in the groove below the next, draw firmly outwards, along the curve of the ribs. Ease pressure toward the shoulders.

CHEST SENSITIVITY

For both men and women, the chest is very erotic, with heightened responses in the nipples and breasts. However, a woman's chest is more sensitive and should be worked around very gently. On a man the pectoral muscles (more accessible on a man than a woman) benefit from releasing massage as they can become quite tight. Here, the massage movements can be performed more broadly, the pectoral muscles circled firmly. Then the movements should be brought in closer, the sensitivity of the touch growing greater as the circles decrease.

3. figure-eight

Supporting with one hand at the shoulder, use your other hand to slide down between your partner's breasts. Continue with a circle around the breast, gliding your hand underneath (far left). Bring your movement round toward the side, and stroking continuously, draw up toward the shoulder (left). Keep your hands sensitive and soft. Then bringing your hand back towards the center, begin to circle the other breast, to make a figure-eight. Change hands if you feel more comfortable and once more glide between the breasts (below, far left). Follow round and under the curve to pull gently up the side (below left). Complete the movement several times. Keep your touch close and softly arousing, then cup your hands around the breasts (main picture). Allow your partner to experience the sensations flowing over her body. These movements are equally as erotic for a woman as for a man.

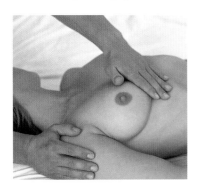
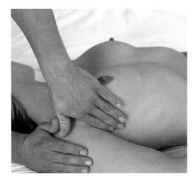
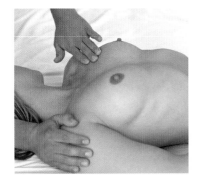
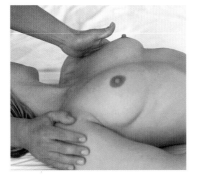

94

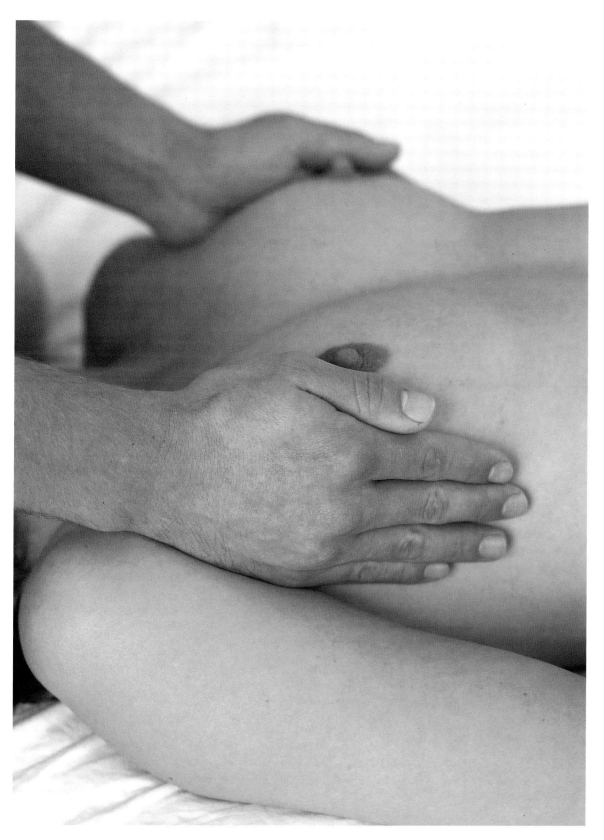

THE ABDOMEN

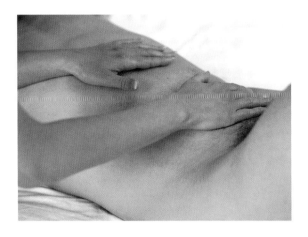

1. effleurage and circling

Cover your hands with more oil. Then approaching contact with your partner sensitively, effleurage, moving your hands in a clockwise direction (above). Let your hands follow the curve of the ribcage. Still circling in the same direction, make your movements a little deeper, pressing with the flat of your hand (below left). As your hands cross over each other, always have one hand continuing the pressure. Leaning over your partner, knead the muscles along his side, pulling and rolling the flesh away from the body (below right). Repeat this movement on the other side, then resume the broad circling with your hands. Expand your circles to tantalize him (main picture).

Moving naturally down from the chest, the strokes to the abdomen are a completion of the torso massage. Look at your partner's body, notice the curves, the angle of the hips and the unprotected nature of the abdomen. Then from the soft, sensual pelvic area, draw your gaze up along your partner's side. Make your first contact by resting your hands lightly in the center of his body.

The abdomen is very sensitive and the quality of your first touch will be immediately felt by your partner. Gentle, warming contact with the flat of the hand feels particularly good in this area. When you massage always move in a clockwise direction (this means you will be following the shape of the large intestine). The lower abdomen is an important area in terms of inner strength, and being centered here affects our vitality. The abdomen can also be affected by nervous tension and anxiety, which results in feeling run down and weak. For this reason, be even more sensitive than usual when massaging the abdomen, and send positive thoughts through your hands. After the

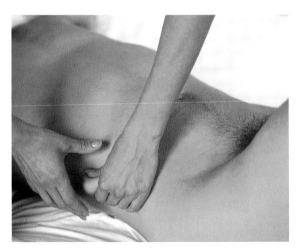

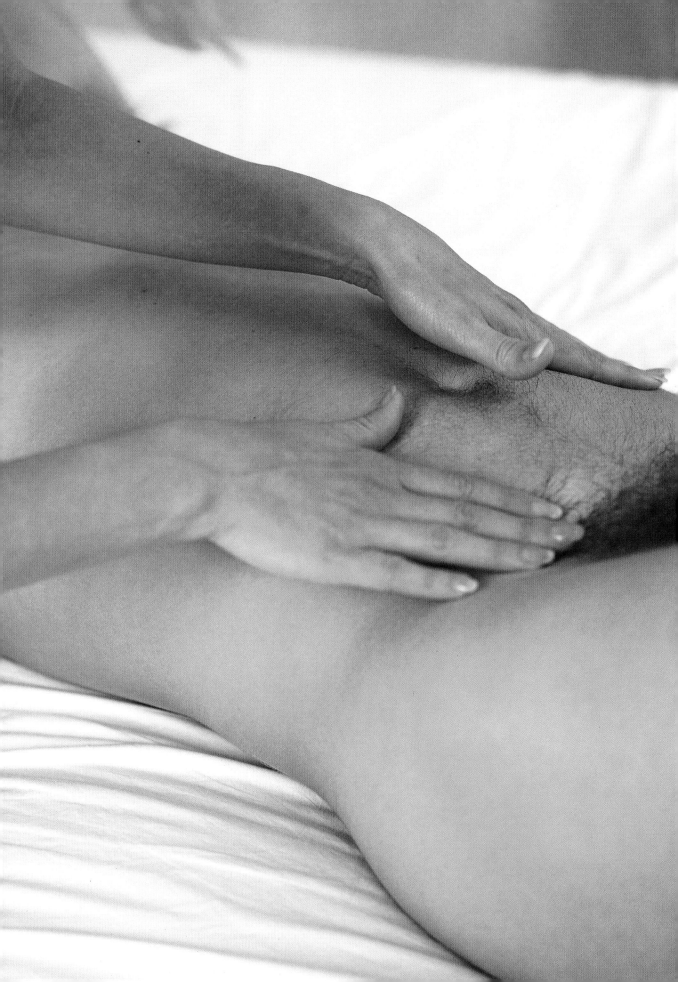

initial effleurage you can continue the circling motion of your hands gradually allowing the pressure to increase. Try and keep the strokes flowing and smooth as your hands cross over each other, expanding the circles slowly to arouse your partner. Knead and pull along your partner's sides, drawing the muscles away from the body. (The large abdominal muscle is the 'external oblique', under which lie layers of muscles which help in flexing the back.) Be careful not to bring the movement into the center. A sideways stretch across the abdomen is good for relieving tension. At the end of the massage softly hold your partner, providing balance, while diffusing the feelings aroused by your strokes. For a man, the abdomen is particularly arousing and sensitive, so keep pressure gentle but firm. For a woman, the area may be quite tender, depending on her menstrual cycle.

As you massage, keep your movements free and sensual, enjoying every tiny bit of your partner's body. The abdomen varies a great deal from person to person. It can be full, round and soft, or muscular and flat. It is a wonderful area for your hands. Notice the skin texture, the way the body curves, the hairs covering the skin, the deep relaxing breaths coming down the torso.

2. stretch and balance

After the circling movements, bring your hands softly to the center of your partner's abdomen and place them together, facing diagonally across the body. Pressing evenly and steadily with the flat of your hands, slowly draw them apart (below). Bring one hand to the hip and the other to the rib cage, caressing the sides of the body. Then repeat this movement in the other direction. Your strokes should be smooth, gliding and continuous. As you end, place one hand over the abdomen and the other softly underneath (main picture). This balances your partner and diffuses the surge of feelings, bringing you and your partner very close. Enjoy watching the way your partner's body moves as he breathes.

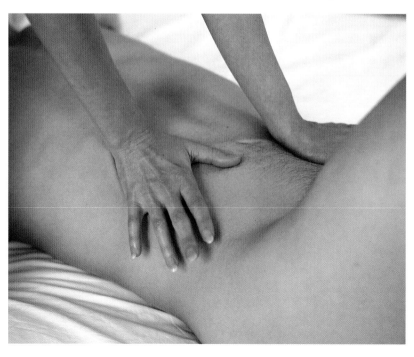

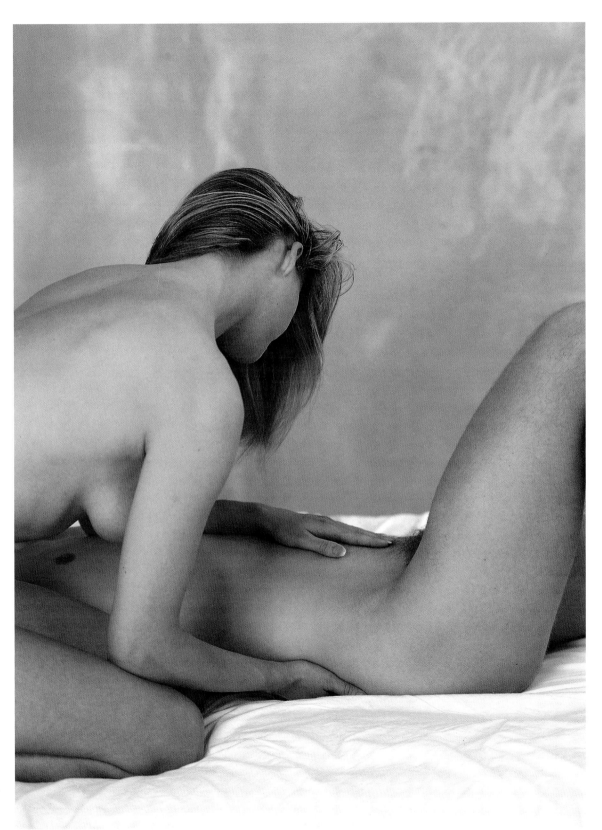

A FULL SENSUAL MASSAGE - *the abdomen*

THE FRONT OF THE LEGS

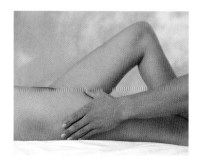

1. effleurage and squeeze

Kneeling at your partner's feet, spread some oil onto your hands, then glide them over her legs (above). Effleurage around the upper thigh and hip. Return to press firmly up the calf muscles either side of the bone (below left). Use your heels for extra pressure. Slide the length of your thumbs around your partner's knee (below right), circling and pressing around its shape. Lifting your partner's thigh, squeeze firmly down the muscles using the heels of the hand to give firmer pressure (main picture). Stroke gently on the inner thigh.

From the tender work on the abdomen, move on to the front of your partner's legs, completing the flow of sensations over the front of the body. Before continuing your contact, look once more at your partner's legs. From the delicate shape of the ankle, to the knees and along the thighs, follow up and over the curve of the hips. Notice how the legs naturally turn out, coming down to the softness of the toes. Make your first contact by resting your hands gently over the top of your partner's feet.

GENERAL POINTS ABOUT MASSAGING THE LEGS
When you begin to effleurage her legs, reach right up over your partner's thighs, bringing your strokes over and around the hips. Remember to rock the legs gently on the downward stroke to loosen the joints and muscles. The pelvis plays an important part in the movement of the leg, for if it is contracted, this alters the way the legs are held. The pelvis can often be thrust back or forwards, which naturally affects the position of the spine. Very often sexual feelings become trapped, cutting off sensations to the legs.

The squeezing stroke that you use in this massage helps to remove waste products from the muscles, and restores the natural flow of energy. Circling lightly round the kneecap releases pressure in the joint, sending pleasurable sensations round the knee. When you come to massaging the thighs, it is worth realizing that they contain some of the most powerful muscles in

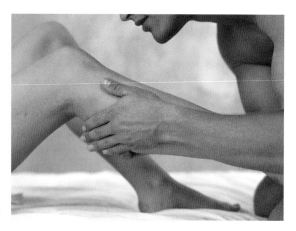

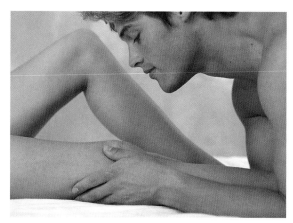

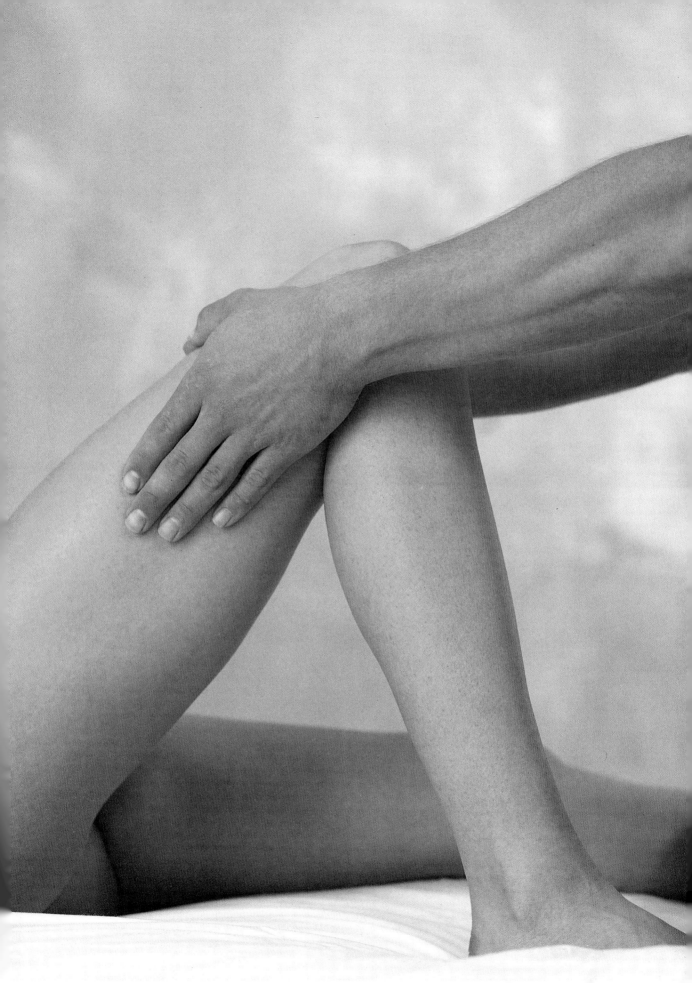

2. pressing and stroking

With your partner's leg still raised, move your hand towards the hip, and press around the hip joint with your fingers (left). Keep the pressure reasonably firm and then press in toward the body, without pressing over the bone. Repeat the movement several times to release tightness around the hips

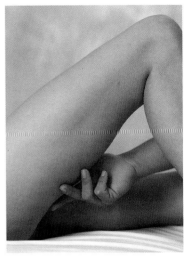

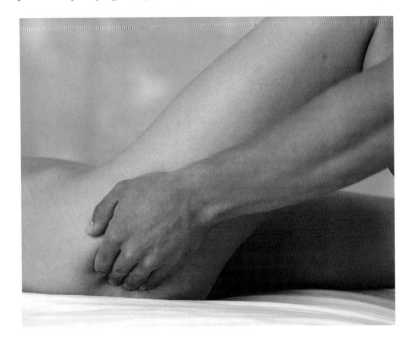

and buttocks. Then softly with your fingertips stroke up the back and inner thigh, heightening the arousal for your partner (above). The delicate strokes over the skin contrast with the movement over the hip, helping to diffuse the strong sensations already aroused.

the body and appreciate firm massage. However, you must ease the pressure as you approach the knee joint. You will also need to change your position so that you can reach down the whole length of the leg. Your partner will absolutely love this.

As you massage, 'listen' to your partner's legs. Try to ascertain where they need attention. If your partner plays a lot of sport, for example, the thighs may be particularly hungry for deep pressure. The feet also enjoy firm pressure, and the ankles, knees and hips benefit from being stretched. Passive movements on the legs feel both liberating and deliciously enjoyable. Giving the entire weight of your body to your partner, let him take responsibility for your limbs. The fronts of your legs

adore sensual strokes, especially light touches down the thighs and around the knees. The front of the feet and ankles are also extremely sensitive, as are the toes. After the stretching movements, tenderly stroke the length of your partner's legs with long strokes and then softly caress the feet. When performing the circling and stretches move close in to your partner and you can then move the joints freely. As you rotate the hip, explore the movement of the joint, without exerting pressure on the knee. The hip joint, like the shoulder, a ball and socket joint, is held firmly in place by strong ligaments. As the joint itself is quite deep, these rolls feel particularly rewarding. Be inventive when massaging the front of your partner's legs, taking full advantage of their flexibility.

Be very sensitive to your partner, and always check that the pressure feels all right. There is a type of pressure that feels as if it is doing good, and there is another, which is simply pain. Massage should never hurt your partner.

ABOUT THE FRONT OF THE LEGS

Along the front of the thighs run the powerful 'quadriceps' muscles, used in hip and knee movements. Crossing the thigh is the 'sartorius' muscle, the longest muscle of the body. The muscles of the calf affect the movements of the ankle as well as being used to extend the toes. When massaging the calves, work to either side of the shins, as it can be painful pressing directly on the bone. Be sensitive

with regard to the knee, which contains thin cartilage between the bones, and while resilient, can sometimes be quite fragile. The knees are also a place where tension is often held. They should remain slightly bent for energy to flow freely.

As well as providing the means for motion, our legs are also our stability. Tension affects the way we stand. When standing, both legs and feet should be relaxed, the feet planted firmly on the ground. You may find that you stand with your toes curled, as if you are gripping on to life. Spend time finding the balance in your stance. Retain an even pressure between the heel and the ball of the foot. Imbalance affects the entire body position.

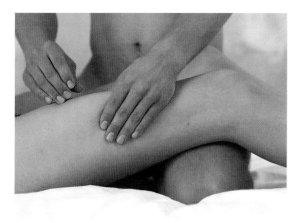

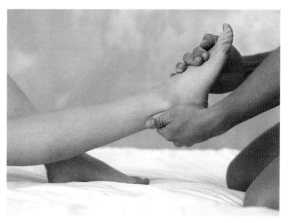

3. kneading and stretching

Rest your partner's thigh over your leg and begin to knead the muscles firmly and deeply (above left). Start the kneading movements at the top of the thigh, gradually working toward the knee. Knead firmly along the front of the leg, rolling the flesh up and away from the bone. In order to deeply penetrate the muscles, use your

thumbs to give extra pressure to the rolls. As the muscles can be quite tight here, keep your wrists flexible to allow the maximum movement of your hands. Ease the pressure as the muscles taper toward the knee. Then lower the leg and move to your partner's feet. Placing one hand around the heel and the other over the foot, lift your partner's leg and pull

slowly back toward you. This stretch reaches along the leg to the hip (above right). Pull back with your arms straight, using the weight of the body, keeping a gradual pressure until you feel resistance. Then, still holding your partner's foot, lower it gently with your hands. Keep support with one hand under the heel and move the other to the knee.

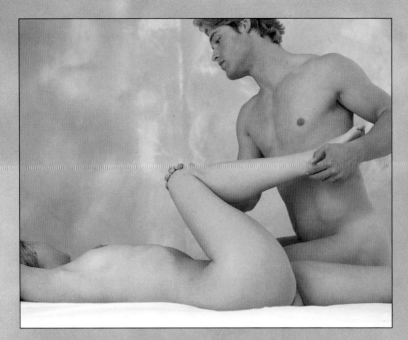

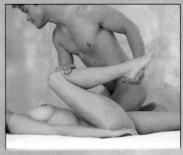

surrendering the weight of her leg.
Press to the point of resistance,
then lower her leg slowly.

4. thigh, hip and lower back

With one hand beneath the foot
and the other at the knee (main
picture) bend your partner's leg
toward her chest. Supporting her
leg, slowly circle it outwards across
her body (above left). You will find
that the hip opens naturally to the
side. The movement affects the
hips and lower back. Then press

your partner's leg toward her
chest, giving a stretch along the
front of the thigh (above right).
Make sure your partner relaxes,

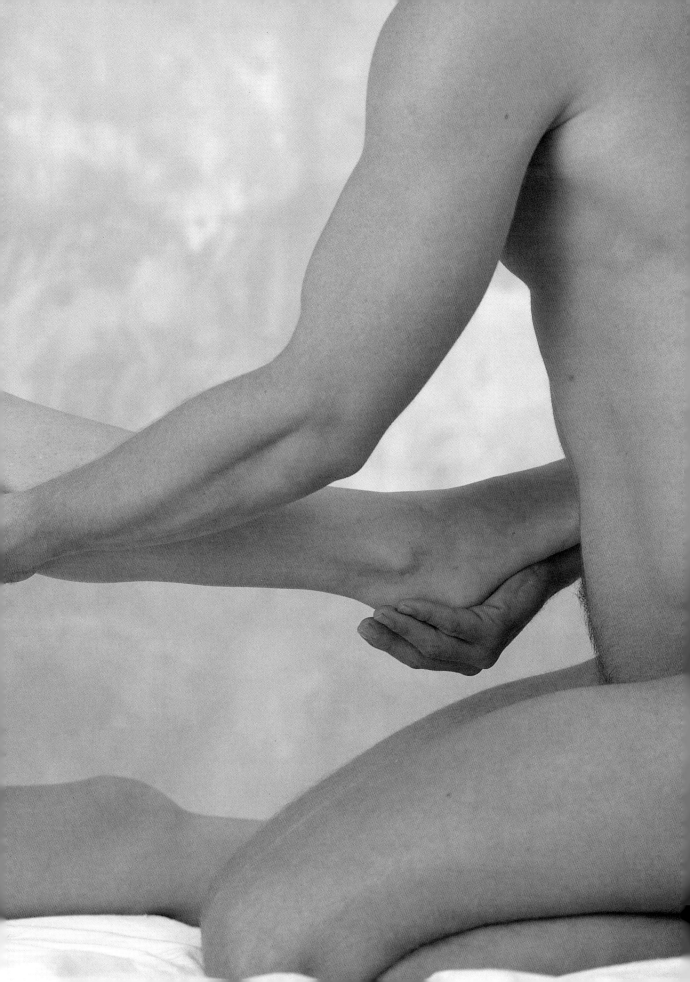

5. opening and pressing

Rest your partner's leg against your thigh, then place the length of your thumbs together across the foot. Cup your fingers under the sole. Pressing upwards with your fingers create an arch, and draw your thumbs over the top of the foot moving outwards from the center (below). Use the heels of your thumbs to draw the tension out, giving the sense of opening and expansion. Repeat this several times over. Supporting the foot, press across the sole with the flat of your thumb (right), pressing in and then withdrawing pressure evenly. Press firmly round the toes and continue the movement over the heel, but reduce the pressure in the fleshy center of the foot.

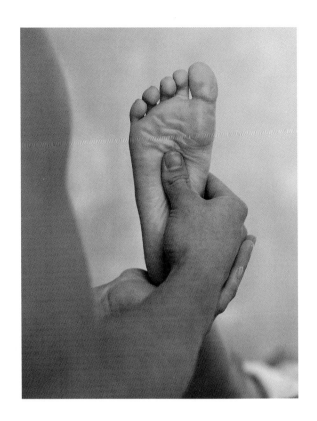

THE FEET

Now turn your attention wholly to your partner's feet. Open out the foot by pressing up and pulling across the bones. This releases the whole foot. (The top of the foot rarely receives much attention). Then press the sole of the foot firmly for deeply relaxing sensations. Hook your fingers around the toes and give little tugs. Firm pressure around the toe joints feels instantly satisfying, easing the pressure around the sensitive instep. As a contrast to the pressure on your partner's foot, hold the foot softly, wrapping your fingers around it, and then simply resting your hands. This focuses awareness down your partner's body, and provides a feeling of stillness.

REFLEXOLOGY

In a reflexology massage various points on the feet (which relate to specific areas of the body) can be massaged to relax and tone its corresponding area of the body. The theory is that the body is divided into zones, so the reflex of an organ or structure will be found in the corresponding zone on the foot. The underside of the foot follows the shape of the body with the line for the diaphragm running just below the ball. The waist line runs across the center of

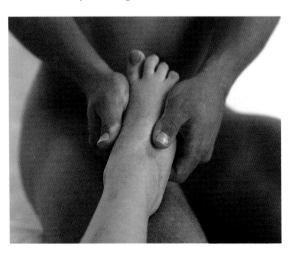

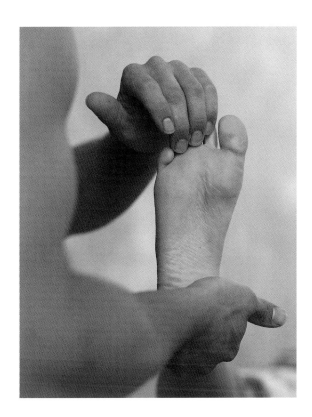

with tender areas designating where tension lies. You may find it valuable to bear these points in mind as you massage your partner's feet. Whatever your movements, be sure your partner will enjoy them.

COMPLETING THE MASSAGE
Spend some time just feeling the sensations between you and your partner, as the feelings flow down your partner's body. All the sensations of the massage are now centered in your partner's feet. Now it is time for soft, gentle caresses and stroking. Your partner will be completely relaxed and at the same time will be experiencing a renewal of her inner vital energy. Spend a little time caressing her feet, pulling and separating the toes. Then draw your hands softly along her feet, perhaps also brushing gently with your lips. Draw the massage to a close keeping contact with your partner's eyes.

One of the most delightful moments of the experience for you will take place as your partner becomes ready for activity. You will soon discover that the pleasure of receiving a massage is highly infectious. Get ready to enjoy this time together.

the foot and the heel line crosses the heel. The various parts of the body are then mapped onto the foot according to their position. For example, the toes contain the reflexes for the head, the kidneys are represented in the center of the foot, and the spinal reflexes run along the inside edge. By pressing the foot you can stimulate a particular part of the body

6. stretch and pull
Still supporting your partner's heel in your hand, curl your fingers underneath her toes (top). Then having hooked them around the foot, gently stretch and pull. You may be able to lift the entire foot and shake the toes gently to loosen any tension. Your partner can curl her toes around your hand. After a few moments, use

gentle brushstrokes down the legs and teasingly bringing your hands down over the foot. Then softly fold your hands around her foot (right), keeping your body completely still. This helps to focus sensations, and draws the energy to your partner's feet. When you feel ready, begin the movement sequence on the other leg. This will bring the massage to a close.

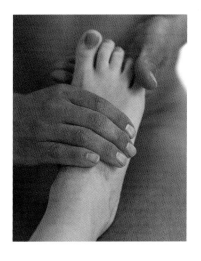

SHARING THE EXPERIENCE

*W*ith *wonderfully pleasurable sensations flowing all over your partner's body, end the massage with lively, light-hearted strokes. Ripple your fingers down the front of your partner's body, tickling and gently teasing her. This will uplift her energy, creating a dynamism between you. Keep the contact constant with your eyes. After lying down for the length of the massage, your partner will probably need a few minutes in order to adjust to movement. When ready she should roll over toward her side, then push herself up into a sitting position with her hand.*

After a massage, whether relaxing or sensual, the whole body feels absolutely sensational, much lighter and infused with a profound sense of general well-being. Smiles and laughter come naturally. Massage reaches to the very heart of a person, creating special moments for two loving people to share.

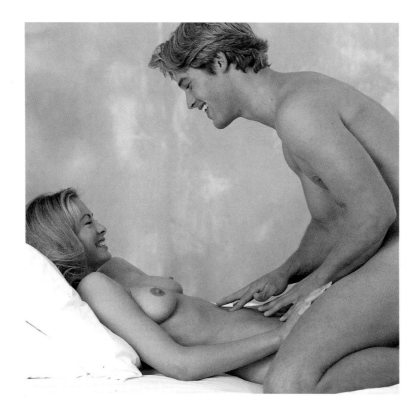

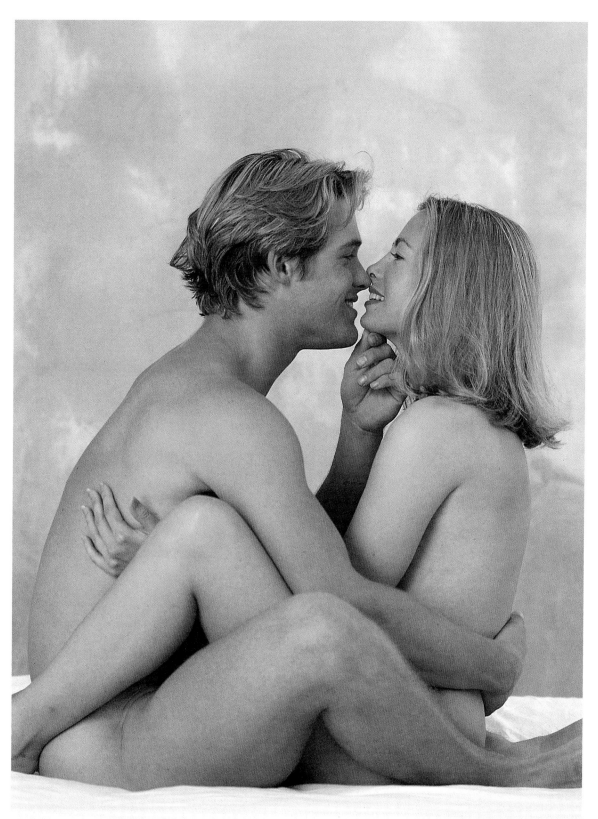

Play after
MASSAGE

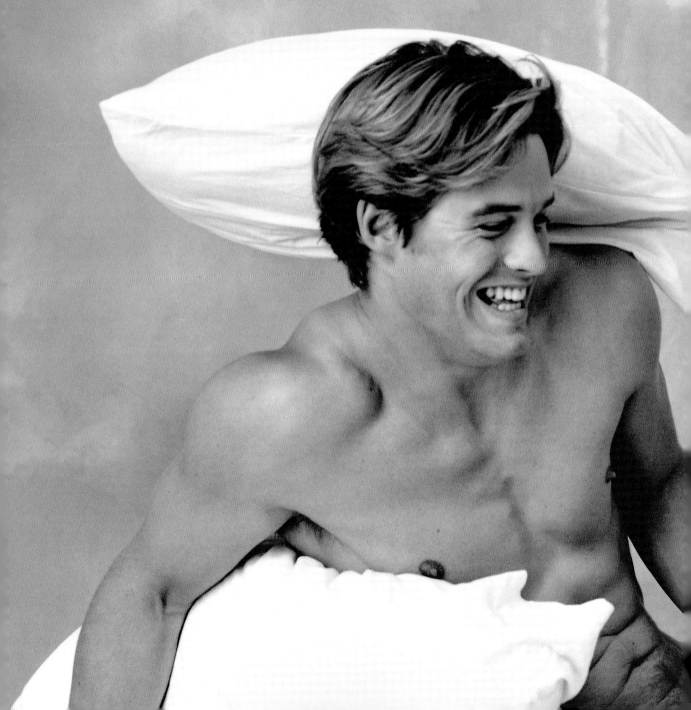

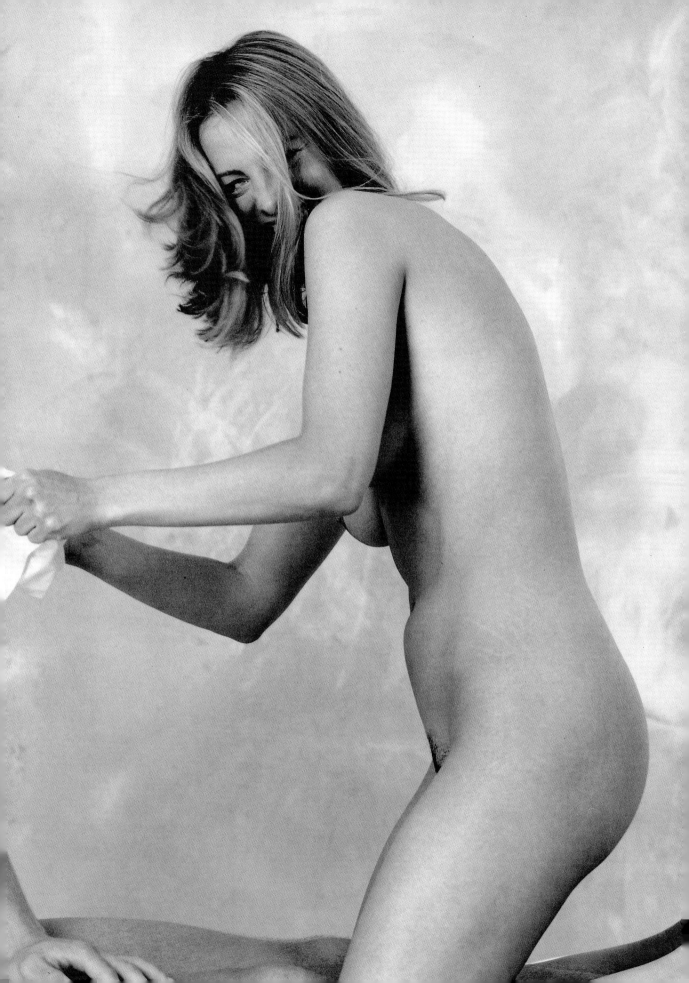

PLAY AFTER MASSAGE

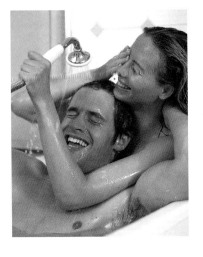

With creativity, you can turn the time you spend follow-ing the massage into a whole new experience. One way to continue your heightened sensuality is to have a bath and luxuriate in the soft feel of water infused with essential oils. Allow a little time for your body to absorb the massage oil and resume its natural rhythm. Bathing with your partner provides an opportunity for tenderness as well as being enormous fun.

Fill your bath with essential oils or a luxurious foam bath preparation. Or as an alternative use a small amount of natural sea salt, which is both cleansing and reviving. Fill your bath-room with things that appeal to your senses, such as sponges, vegetable soaps, and scented shampoos. Water is soft, cleansing and sensual – immerse yourself in it.

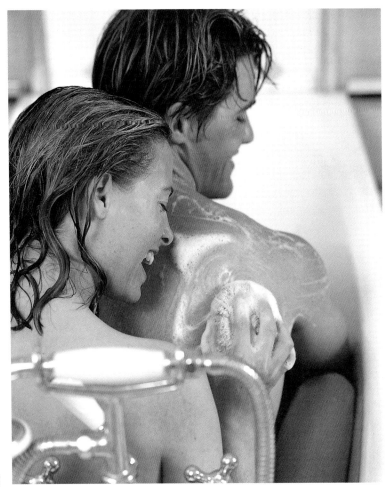

creative cleansing

Use a soft natural sponge to soap your partner's body with a pure vegetable soap, gel or cream (left). Rub thoroughly over the skin, working in small circles to help slough off any dead skin cells. Starting on the back, soap all over your partner's body. It feels wonderful and leaves the skin stimulated and vibrant. Use a soft hand-shower to rinse off any soap, or to lightly sprinkle water all over the body (above). The wetter you both get, the better, and this way, you can have a shower and a bath at once! It also feels good to shampoo your partner's hair, giving the scalp a good massage as you do so. Afterwards gently stroke her hair as you hold her, enjoying the wetness of her body (main picture). Your partner will be enveloped by your tender attention.

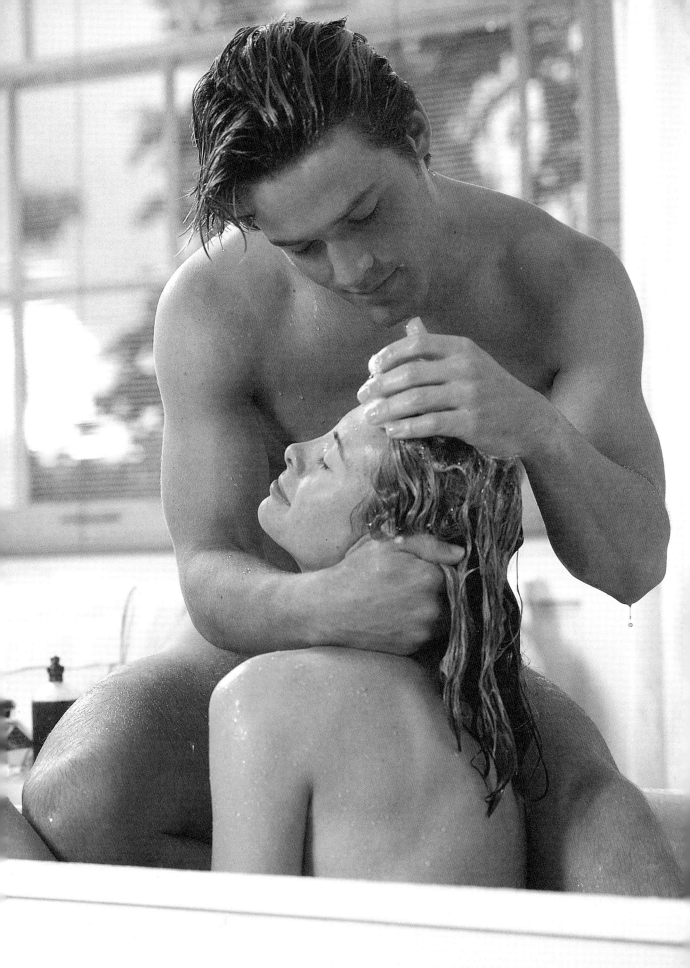

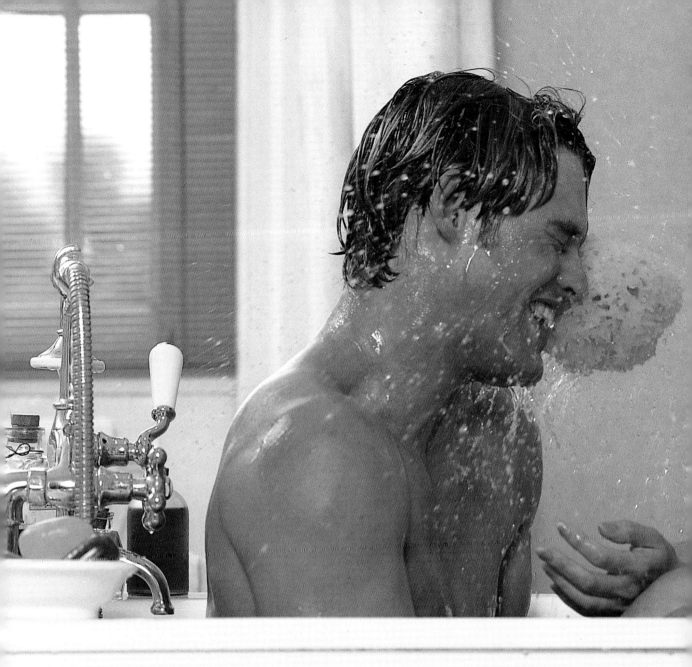

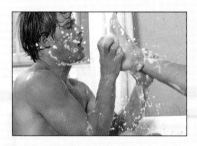
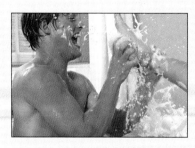
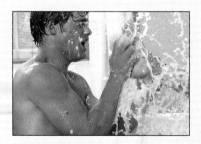

fun in the bath

In the bath, let go. Flick each other
with water to get each other totally
wet or to see if you can score a
direct hit! The sheer freedom
and the feel of water encourages
playfulness and a delight in being
childish. Soaping your partner's
leg is not necessarily an easy
business, even if you put your
whole heart into it. Use a sponge
or face cloth to soap the length of

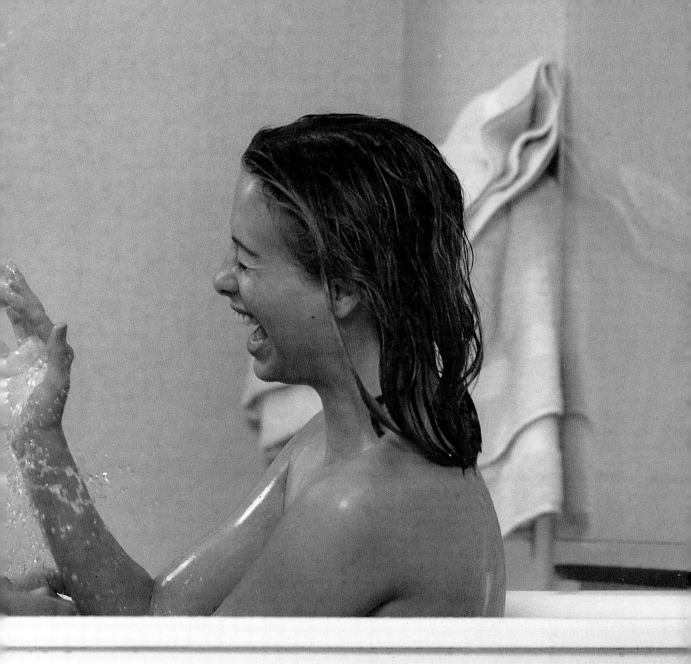

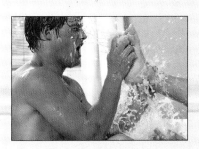 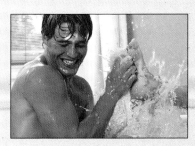 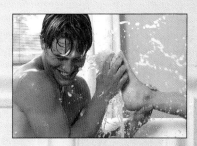

her leg, using long, soapy strokes right up along her thigh. This feels incredibly sensual as well as being great fun. Make sure you soap

over your partner's foot and slide in between the toes. Afterwards, give your partner a warm, wet foot massage, scrubbing over the

sole as vigorously as you dare. It is vital to the life of the relationship to simply let go and enjoy each other.

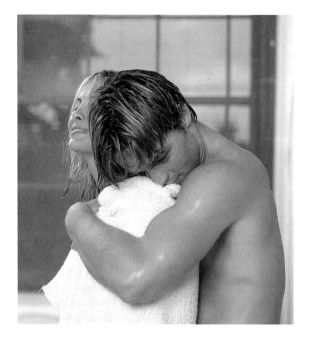

gentle drying

Use a soft, warm towel to wrap right around your partner, and then carefully dry every inch of her. Holding the towel over her, rub through the material to bring a warm glow to her skin.

This action feels very comforting. It is an expression of great tenderness to perform these simple actions for another person. You can take the opportunity to hug your partner and hold her very close.

AFTER BATHING

Continue the feelings by making towelling after the bath a wonderful sensual experience. Use huge, soft, warmed towels to wrap around each other and pat each other's bodies dry. Taking care of each other in these very basic ways creates tremendous feelings of warmth and intimacy. To prevent your skin from drying, use a thin covering of lotion or oils. Adding some essential oils, you can make various preparations for either relaxation, sensuality or stimulation. A particularly refreshing combination is a mixture of lavender and rosemary oil (see pages 122-123). Rub the oils over your partner's body, making sure they sink into the skin. For an interesting variation, rub the oil in with your feet.

Afterwards, stimulate your partner through some invigorating massage movements. These have a completely different effect from the previous movements as they are used to tone and stimulate the body. While using the strokes of conventional western massage, this stimulating massage is based on the eastern acupressure approach. The idea is to stimulate meridians along the body, along which the path of energy flows. There are 14 meridians, relating to organs of the body, incorporating the mind and emotions. When a pathway becomes blocked, disease arises. Keeping the channels clear keeps the body in balance.

Once again you will be working from the upper body to the feet. Your partner will need to be standing or seated. Pummel with loose fists along the top of the back, working toward the spine from the edge of the shoulder. Use your fists alternately in short, pounding movements, going backwards and forwards several times. Stop just short of the spine. The looser your wrists, the better the action feels. Perform the movements along the other shoulder, then change your action slightly. With your fingers held loosely together, use the edges of your hands to make hacking movements over the top of the shoulder. Keep loose, flexible wrists in fast alternating movements, making contact

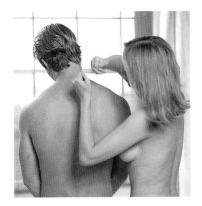

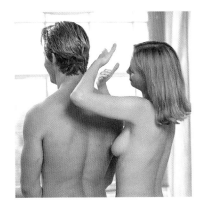

working the shoulders

Closing your hands into loose fists, pummel across the top of the shoulders (top). Work toward the neck, stopping in the angle formed with the spine. Repeat on the opposite shoulder, then use the edges of your hands alternately to make light hacking movements (above).

with the line of your little fingers. As you use your hands, your fingers will flick against each other. The actions should remain sharp but light, feeling particularly good in the angle between the shoulder and the spine. Repeat the movement again on the other shoulder. Then cupping your hands, move to your partner's arms, and cup down the arms from the shoulders to the wrists. This movement stimulates sensations in the arms, and leaves a lively tingling feeling in the hands. Your actions should feel good and enjoyable. After completing the movements several times on both arms, bend down to stimulate your partner's legs. Using light movements with your fists, first pat up the inside of the leg, then over the top of the thigh, finishing down the outside of the leg. Use the underside of your fists, making contact with the fingers. This movement should be light and invigorating, and brings the sensations down to your partner's feet. After performing the movements on the other leg, the entire body should feel alive and stimulated.

Massage can reach the body in a new way. Using the different strokes you have learnt and working at different speeds not only firms and tones the muscles, it also activates and alerts the body and mind. The intention of the massage also makes a difference to your partner, and greatly alters the way you will perform the strokes. Our bodies have an amazing store of secrets that can be tapped, and are greatly influenced by our interactions. Moving over the body in different ways produces different results. Follow your intuition and let your feelings guide you as you massage. Listen to the responses of your partner. The body knows if it needs to be relaxed, stimulated or simply stroked and hugged.

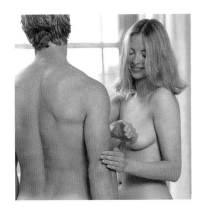

the limbs

Cupping yor hands over the arm, pat vigorously from the shoulder to the wrist (left). Work down the outside of each arm, then use the underside of your fists to tap up the inside of the legs. Work over the thigh and down the outer side to the ankle (right).

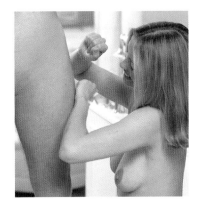

Now your muscles are toned and you are feeling energetic, ease into some active body movements with your partner. Mutual massage is always fun to do as well as being beneficial. Sitting on the floor, press against your soles to massage each other's feet. Use the heel, toes and ball of your feet to cover as wide an area as possible. Turning your feet sideways, you can massage each other's feet. Be inventive. The more you use your legs, the better the massage feels. Then, turning back to back, try a mutual back massage. This probably works best if one person is active at a time. Again be inventive, slide and wriggle up and down your partner's back, massaging with your shoulders as far down as you can. Your partner should resist by pressing against you. This always feels fantastic, and is impossible to do without dissolving into laughter.

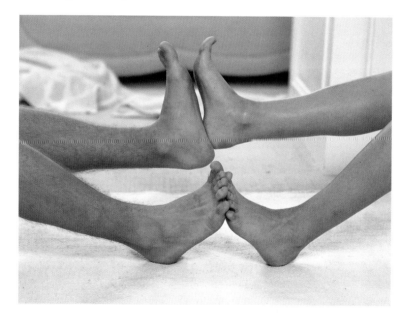

mutual massage magic

Sitting facing each other, with your arms behind you for support, place the soles of your feet together. Then move and press over the soles of each other's feet, including the toes and heels (above). Both press at the same time. Have your heels on the ground to give support. Then back to back, one of you massages the other by pressing with your shoulders up and down your partner's back (main picture). Using your arms for support, slide down as far as you can, while your partner provides resistance against you.

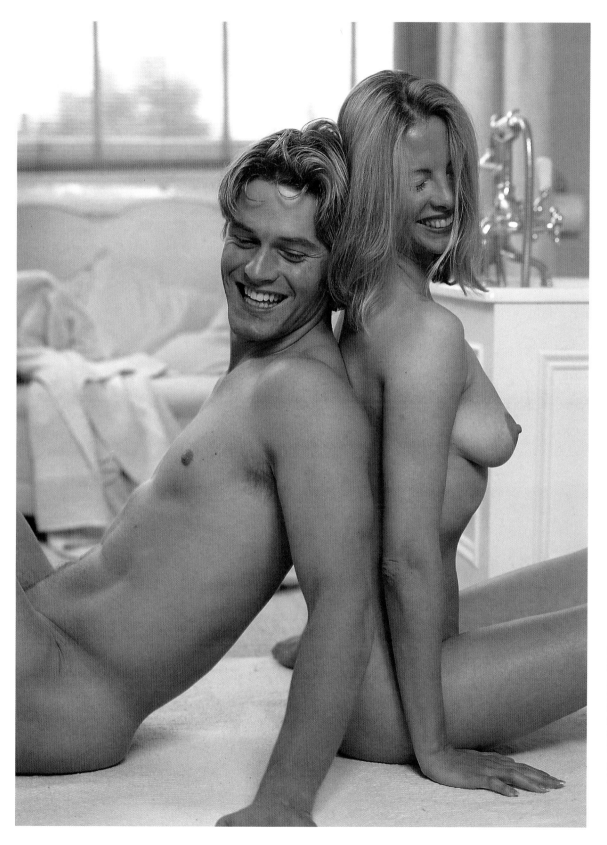

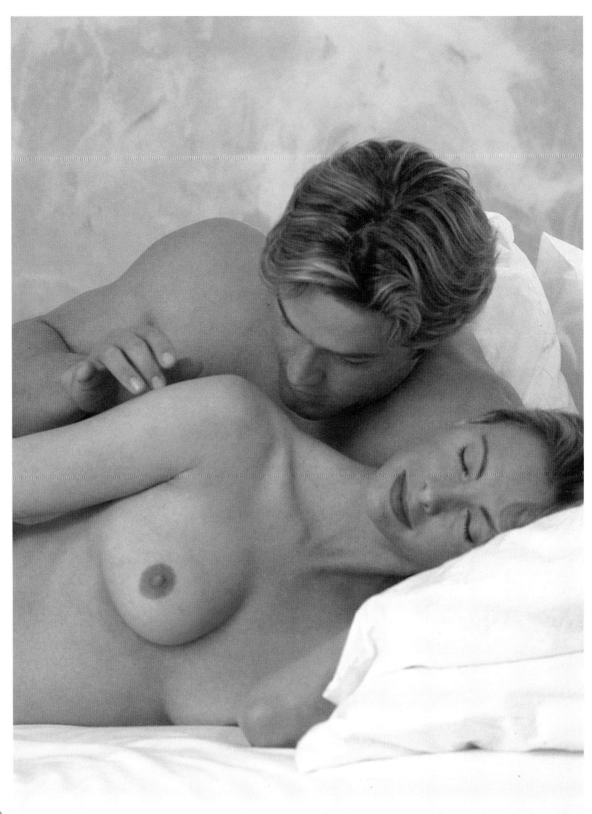

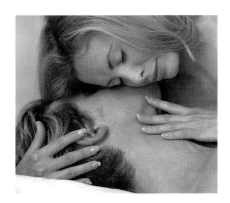

Sensual Tips

After bathing, oiling and massaging, continue with sensual creativity. Allow the opportunitites for sensual experience to go on and on. Run a comb through your partner's hair and watch the way the hair reacts. Trickle oil or water down your partner's body and watch the movement and the qualities of liquid running over skin. Or use a wooden massage roller over your partner's thigh as an alternative sensation to your hands. You could experiment with the sensations of various foods and drinks and the feel of different materials on the skin. Or just feel the sensations produced as you lie together, noticing each other's breath and warmth.

Discover the magic in our everyday activities and surroundings. Not only are the senses fundamental to the enjoyment of our relationships, but through release and revitalization, they inspire our work. By focusing on sensuality in our lives, we keep both mind and body healthy.

Touching through sensual massage maintains a fresh, rich, rewarding relationship. It gives us an opportunity to find out about each other, to give in an extraordinarily beautiful way. Our partner becomes more familiar, and yet somehow more mysterious. It is also, in the end, a way of giving to ourselves as the benefits enhance and strengthen our relationship. Learning to give a massage is an invaluable gift, a precious exchange of intimacy. As you learn about your partner, so your skills increase, and your enjoyment grows. The partnership is strengthened by caring practically for each other with a new understanding that defies definition.

121

OILS AND THEIR USES

A brief guide to some useful essential oils and their health-giving properties and qualities.

BASIL
Antiseptic. Nerve tonic. Uplifts. (Avoid during pregnancy.)

BERGAMOT
Antiseptic. Good for skin and respiratory infections. Sedative, Uplifting. (Avoid using neat on skin or in direct sunlight.)

CHAMOMILE
Soothes inflammation. Relieves aches and pains and dry skin. Sedative. Anti-depressant.

CLARY SAGE
Nerve tonic. Sedative. Good for nervous depression. Helps ease painful periods. Promotes childbirth. Aphrodisiac.

FRANKINCENSE
Astringent. Relieves catarrh. Soothing. Rejuvenating.

GERANIUM
Skin cleanser and tonic. Mild diuretic. Sedative. Uplifting.

JASMINE
Sedative. Anti-depressant. Anti-spasmodic. Relieves period pains. Promotes childbirth. Euphoric. Aphrodisiac.

JUNIPER
Nerve tonic. Astringent and skin tonic. Diuretic. Relieves indigestion. Sedative.

LAVENDER
Antiseptic. Relieves skin inflammation and burns. Relieves stomach complaints. Sedative. Relaxing. The most useful all-round oil.

MARJORAM
Nerve tonic. Aids digestion. Relieves muscle spasm. Lowers blood pressure. (Avoid using during pregnancy.)

MELISSA
Tonic. Anti-depressant. Relieves hysteria and palpitations. Regulates menstrual cycle. Uplifting.

NEROLI
Regenerates the skin. Relieves diarrhoea. Sedative. Anti-depressant. Calming. Aphrodisiac.

PATCHOULI
Stimulant. Astringent. Aids mental clarity. Aphrodisiac.

ROSE
Antiseptic. Cleansing. Soothing. Promotes circulation. Strengthens digestive system. Relieves stress. Good for mature, dry skin. Aphrodisiac.

ROSEMARY
Antiseptic. Stimulant. Aids mental clarity. Heart tonic. Clears dandruff. Cleansing. Relieves headaches as well as general aches and pains.

SAGE
Nerve tonic. Diuretic. Relieves general aches and pains.

SANDALWOOD
Relieves dry, inflamed skin, sore throats and coughs. Sedative. Aphrodisiac.

THYME
Antiseptic. Nerve tonic. Relieves headaches and general aches and pains. Stimulates circulation. Invigorating.

YLANG YLANG
Lowers blood pressure. Good for oily skin. Aphrodisiac. Sedative. Euphoric. (Use only in small quantities.)

Fill a 1 floz (28ml) bottle three quarters full
with grapeseed oil.
Add five per cent almond oil.
Add half a teaspoon of wheat germ oil for
preservation (optional).
Add 12 drops of essential oil.
Fill up the remainder of the bottle with
grapeseed oil.
Use a screw-top bottle and store in
a cool place.

Recipes for 1floz (28ml) of oil

RELAXING MASSAGE OIL
*Mix seven drops of lavender and five drops of
chamomile to the base massage oil
or simply 12 drops of lavender*

THREE SENSUAL MASSAGE OILS
*To the base massage oil you can add
eight drops of ylang ylang and
four drops of neroli
or eight drops of sandalwood with four
drops of ylang ylang
or six drops of jasmine with six drops of rose*

RELAXATION AFTER-BATHING OIL
*Add eight drops of lavender and four drops of
geranium to a base oil made up of 1floz (28ml) of
almond oil with five per cent avocado oil added*

SENSUAL AFTER-BATHING OIL
*Add seven drops of rose and five drops of neroli to
the base oil*

STIMULATING AFTER-BATHING OIL
*Add seven drops of lavender and five drops of
rosemary to the base oil*

MASSAGE CHECK LIST
Oils
Towels
Pillows and cushions
Tissues
Space to move around your partner
Heating
Soft lighting
Some water
Music (optional)
Answering machine
An hour when you will not be disturbed

THE DO'S AND DON'TS OF MASSAGE
As long as you are sensitive and careful, you
will not be able to do any harm at all through
massage. However, here are a few simple
guidelines to help you:

• Remember to remove any jewelry before you
start a massage and to keep your nails reasonably short.
• Do not massage after a heavy meal or have a
hot bath afterwards.
• Do not try to cure persistant muscular aches
or pains. If your partner has any problems or
experiences any sharp pains during the massage,
consult your doctor or a qualified practitioner.
• Do not massage directly on the spine.
• Do not massage recent injuries.

Traditionally do not massage
• If your partner has a heart condition.
• Over the abdomen in the first four months of
pregnancy.
• Around or over a tumor.
• Over varicose veins.

Always consult your doctor if in doubt.

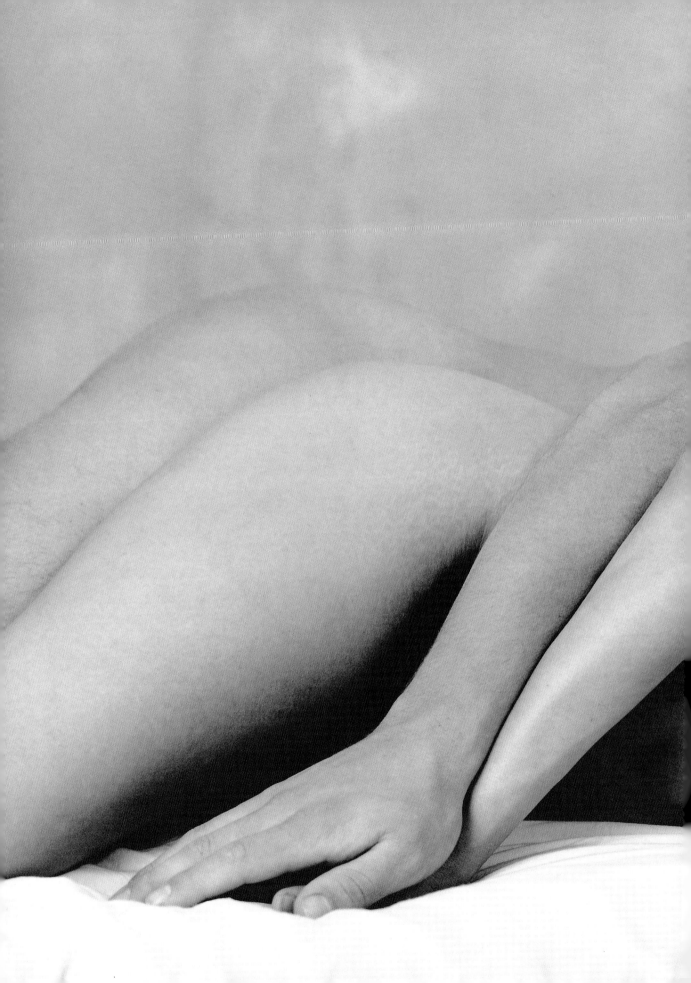

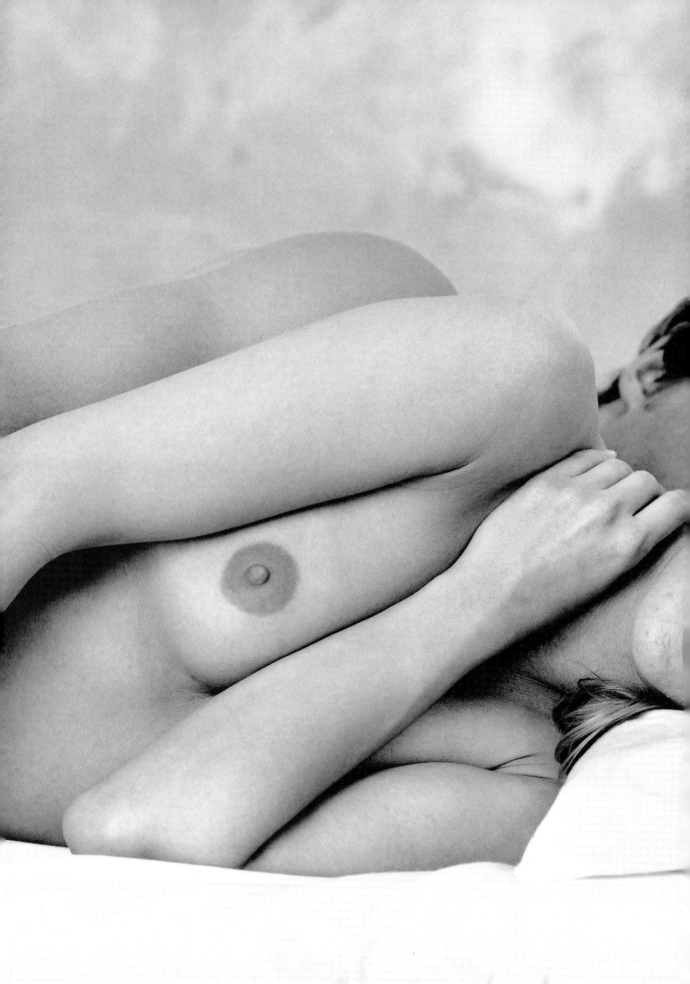

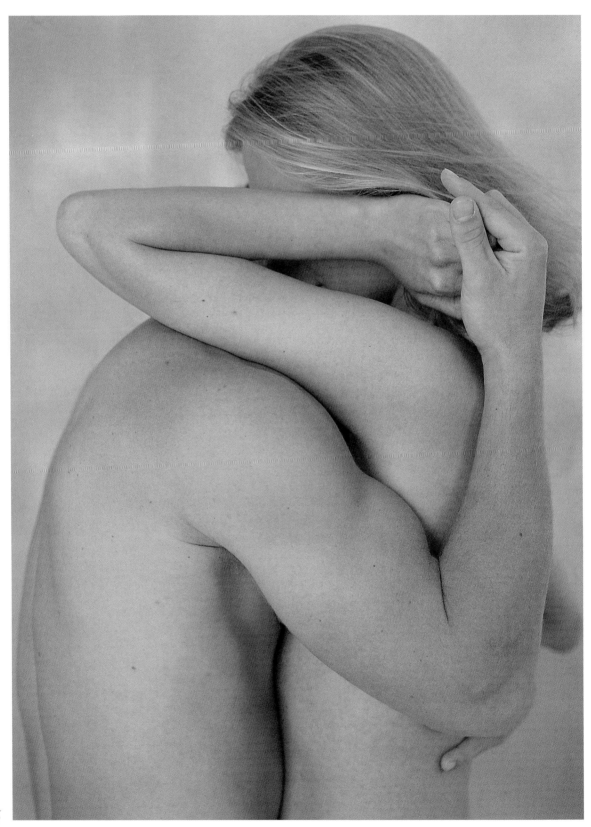

INDEX

ABOUT THE AUTHOR

Susan Mumford is a qualified massage practitioner. She has had a private holistic massage practice in London for several years, and teaches introductory massage and one-to-one relaxation. Susan is trained in healing and counselling, and is also a qualified aromatherapist. She pracises T'ai Chi and meditation to help her work. Her previous books, published by Hamlyn, are *A Complete Guide To Massage* (1995), and *Healing Massage* (1997).

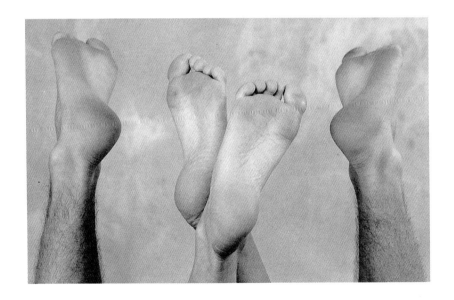

ACKNOWLEDGEMENTS

I would like to thank Dave, Andy, Elizabeth and Neil for their help.
And I would also like to thank my
teachers, and of course, my massage clients.